An Emera

EXPLAINING ARTHRITIS

LIVING WITH AND CONTROLLING ARTHRITIS

Ellen Baxendale

Editor: Roger Sproston

Emerald Guides
www.straightforwardco.co.uk

Emerald Guides

© Straightforward Co Ltd 2019

ISBN 978-1-84716-967-9

Printed by 4edge Ltd www.4edge.co.uk

Cover design by BW Studio Derby

Contents

Introduction

Chapter 1.   6
What is Arthritis and what are its effects ?

Chapter 2.   22
Osteoarthritis

Chapter. 3.   37
Rheumatoid Arthritis

Chapter. 4.   51
Ankylosing Spondylitis and Enteropathic arthritis

Chapter. 5.   62
Cervical Spondylitis

Chapter 6.   71
Fibromyalgia

Chapter 7.   84
Lupus

Chapter 8.   94
Gout

Chapter 9.   101
Psoriatic Arthritis

Chapter 10   **106**
Reactive Arthritis

Chapter 11   **118**
Polymyalgia Rheumatica

Chapter 12   **126**
Juvenile Idiopathic Arthritis

Chapter 13   **132**
The importance of Diet and exercise

Index

****

Introduction

Everyone has heard of arthritis, and knows someone with the condition. However, if we ourselves are not affected by the condition we tend not to know much about it. Arthritis is a common condition that causes joint inflammation and pain, and it affects about 10 million people in the UK. People of all ages can get it and there are many forms of the condition such as Osteoarthritis, Rheumatoid Arthritis and Gout

Being diagnosed with arthritis can raise many questions. This book will provide you with the information you need to understand this condition in all its different forms, the treatment options available to you, different methods of coping, and where to go for further advice and help. It will also, importantly, help you see the 'wood from the trees' and avoid the many offers of treatment in the form of pills and potions that seek to exploit the sufferer.

Diet and exercise are also important elements in the control of arthritis and in chapter 13 we go into both areas in depth.

There is a lot of information around concerning all of the different forms of arthritis. There are good websites around, such as Versus Arthritis (formerly Arthritis UK and Arthritis Research). Also, the NHS website is very good and comprehensive. However, the advantage of a book such as Explaining Arthritis, apart from usefulness to those who do not have or cannot use a computer, is that all of the disparate strands of information are pulled together which can then be used as a reference guide. I hope that you find this introduction useful and of benefit.

Chapter 1

What is Arthritis and What are its Effects ?

Arthritis generally

In this chapter we will provide an overview of the condition known as Arthritis, of which Osteoarthritis and Rheumatoid arthritis are the two most common types. There are about 100 different identified types of arthritis and, obviously, we can't cover them all. The approach we take in this book is to initially discuss each of 12 areas generally and then, chapter by chapter, expand on these areas, with illustrations, and also outline the treatments available. We also outline self-help options and provide a list of useful support groups which can offer further advice. The areas covered are as follows:

- Osteoarthritis
- Rheumatoid arthritis
- Ankylosing spondylitis and Enteropathic arthritis
- Cervical spondylitis
- Fibromyalgia
- Lupus
- Gout
- Psoriatic arthritis
- Reactive arthritis
- Polymyalgia rheumatica
- Juvenile idiopathic arthritis (JIA)

What is Arthritis? A Generald Definition

The word arthritis is used to describe pain, swelling and stiffness in a joint or joints. Around 10 million people in the UK are thought to have arthritis. Arthritis is a common disease and one of the consequences of aging and also living on a cold and wet Island. It can affect people of all ages – even children and teenagers. Some forms of arthritis are more common in older people. We will be discussing arthritis in children a little later in the book.

Although there's no absolute cure for arthritis, (notwithstanding claims to the contrary, particularly by peddlers of various creams and potions) treatments have improved greatly in recent years and, for many types of arthritis, particularly inflammatory arthritis, there's a clear benefit in starting treatment at an early stage.

It may be difficult to say what has caused arthritis. There are several factors that can increase the risk of each type of arthritis. It could be that the genes inherited from your parents or grandparents made you more likely to get arthritis. It can be where you live, lifestyle and so on. The important thing is to get help at a very early stage, by first seeing a doctor.

Arthritis can make life difficult by causing pain and making it harder to get about. The symptoms of arthritis can vary from week to week, and even from day to day. Many types, such as osteoarthritis and rheumatoid arthritis, are long-term conditions.

Looking at joint pain (see diagram overleaf of a normal joint)

7

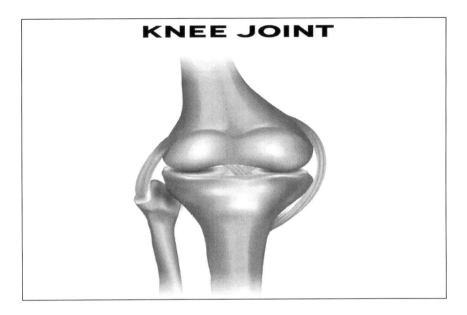

A joint is, simply, where two or more bones meet, such as in the fingers, knees, and shoulders. The above diagram shows a healthy knee joint. Joints hold bones in place and allow them to move freely within limits. Most of the joints in our body are surrounded by a strong capsule. The capsule is filled with a thick fluid that helps to lubricate the joint. These capsules hold our bones in place. They do this with the help of ligaments.

The ends of the bones within a joint are lined with cartilage. This is a smooth but tough layer of tissue that allows bones to glide over one another as you move. If we want to move a bone, our brain gives a signal to the muscle, which then pulls a tendon, and this is attached to the bone. Muscles therefore have an important role in supporting a joint.

As discussed previously, we will expand on the most common types of arthritis chapter by chapter. The below covers a brief outline of the main types of arthritis.

Because there are several types of arthritis, it's important to know which one you have. There are some similarities between these conditions, but there are also some key differences.

Osteoarthritis

The most common type of arthritis, both in the UK and elsewhere in the world, is osteoarthritis. Osteoarthritis starts with the roughening of cartilage. If this happens, the body can put in place a 'repair' process to try to make up for the loss of this important substance. The following can then happen:

- Tiny bits of extra bone, called osteophytes, can grow at the ends of a bone within a joint.
- There can be an increase in the amount of thick fluid inside the joint.
- The joint capsule can stretch, and the joint may lose its shape.

Sometimes, the early stages of osteoarthritis can happen without causing much pain or trouble. However, it can lead to damage inside a joint, as well as pain and stiffness. Osteoarthritis is more common in women and usually affects people from the age of 45 onwards. The parts of the body most commonly affected are the knees, hands, hips, and back. See Chapter 2 for more about Osteoarthritis.

Rheumatoid arthritis

Rheumatoid arthritis is a type of inflammatory arthritis. It is what is known as an auto-immune condition. The immune system is the body's natural self-defence system, and it protects us from infections and illness. When someone has an auto-immune condition, the body's immune system mistakenly attacks the body's healthy tissues, such as the joints, causing inflammation.

Inflammation is normally an important tool in the immune system. It occurs when the body sends extra blood and fluid to an area to fight an infection. This is what is happening for example if you have a cut that gets infected, and the skin around it becomes swollen and a different colour. However, in rheumatoid arthritis the inflammation and extra fluid in a joint can cause the following problems:

- It can make moving the joint difficult and painful.
- Chemicals in the fluid can damage the bone and joint.
- The extra fluid can stretch the joint capsule. Whenever a joint capsule is stretched, it never quite returns to its original position.
- Chemicals in the fluid can irritate nerve endings, which can be painful.

As well as causing pain and stiffness, inflammation can cause permanent damage to a joint. Starting effective treatment early on can help to minimise damage. Symptoms of rheumatoid arthritis can include:

- swollen and tender joints
- swelling and stiffness in joints in the morning that lasts for longer than half an hour
- severe tiredness, also called fatigue
- a general feeling of being unwell.

Rheumatoid arthritis can affect adults of any age. It most commonly starts among people between the ages of 40 and 60.

It's more common in women than men. See chapter 3 for more about Rheumatoid Arthritis.

Spondylosis

Spondyloarthritis is a word used to describe a number of conditions that cause pain and swelling, mainly around the joints of the spine. In these conditions there is inflammation of small pieces of connective tissues, called entheses. These are tough little cords that join either ligaments or tendons to bones.

Ankylosing spondylitis

Ankylosing spondylitis is a type of spondyloarthritis and it causes pain and swelling, mainly around the joints of the spine. In this condition, in response to inflammation around the spine, the body can create more of the mineral calcium. This mineral is normally used by the body to make bones strong. However, in ankylosing spondylitis the extra calcium can make new bits of bone grow in the spine, and this will cause pain and stiffness.

This condition typically causes pain in the second half of the night, and swelling of your back in the morning that lasts for more than half an hour. Ankylosing spondylitis usually occurs between the ages of 20 and 30. It is more common among men.

Cervical spondylitis

Cervical spondylosis is a common, age-related condition that affects the joints and discs in your cervical spine, which is in your neck. It's also known as cervical osteoarthritis or neck arthritis. It develops from the wear and tear of cartilage and bones. While it's largely the result of age, it can be caused by other factors as well.

Some people who have it never experience symptoms. For others, it can cause chronic, severe pain and stiffness. However, many people who have it are able to conduct normal daily activities. See chapters 4 and 5 for more about Spondylitis.

Fibromyalgia

Fibromyalgia is a long-term condition that can cause pain and tenderness all over the body. Symptoms can be similar to arthritis. However, the symptoms are mainly in the muscles rather than the joints. The most common symptoms of fibromyalgia are:

- widespread pain
- trouble sleeping
- fatigue
- headaches
- difficulty concentrating
- a poor memory.

If you have fibromyalgia, you're probably very sensitive to pain or physical pressure. See Chapter 6 for more about Fibromyalgia.

Lupus

Lupus is an auto-immune condition. The immune system mistakenly attacks the body's own healthy tissues. There can be many symptoms of lupus. It's possible for the heart, lungs and other organs of the body to be affected. Joint pain and swelling is common in lupus, particularly in the small joints of the hands and feet. Joint pain in lupus can move around from one joint to another. Lupus can be difficult to diagnose, as it can cause many different symptoms which often appear like other conditions. See Chapter 7 for more about Lupus.

Gout and calcium crystal diseases

Gout is a type of inflammatory arthritis that can cause painful swelling in joints. It typically affects the big toe, but it can also affect other joints in the body. Joints affected by gout can become red and hot. The skin may also look shiny and can peel. It's caused by having too much urate, otherwise known as uric acid, in the body. We all have a certain amount of urate in our body.

However, being overweight or eating and drinking too much of certain types of food and alcoholic drinks can cause some people to have more urate in their bodies. The genes you inherit can make you more likely to develop gout. If it reaches a high level, urate can form into crystals that remain in and around the joint. They can be there for a while without causing any problems and even without the person realising they are there. A knock to a part of the body or having a fever can lead to the crystals falling into the soft part of the joint. This will cause pain and swelling. See Chapter 8 for more about Gout.

Psoriatic arthritis

Psoriatic arthritis is an auto-immune condition. It is also a type of spondyloarthritis. The body's immune system can cause painful swelling and stiffness within and around joints, as well as a red scaly skin rash called psoriasis. The rash can affect several places in the body, including the elbows, knees, back, buttocks and scalp. It is also common to have severe tiredness, otherwise known as fatigue. See Chapter 9 for more about Psoriatic Arthritis.

Reactive arthritis

The most common symptom of reactive arthritis is pain, stiffness and swelling in the joints and tendons, most commonly the knees, feet, toes, hips and ankles. In some people it can also affect the:

- genital tract – causing pain when peeing, or discharge from the penis or vagina
- eyes – causing eye pain, redness, sticky discharge, conjunctivitis and, rarely, inflammation of the eye (iritis)

This could be a symptom of iritis – and the sooner you get treatment, the more successful it is likely to be. Most people will not get all the above symptoms. They can come on suddenly but usually start to develop a few days after you get an infection somewhere else in your body. Typically, reactive arthritis is caused by a sexually transmitted infection, such as chlamydia, or an infection of the bowel, such as food poisoning.

See Chapter 10 for more about Reactive Arthritis.

Polymyalgia rheumatica (PMR)

Polymyalgia rheumatica (PMR) is a condition involving painful and stiff muscles. The hips, shoulders and thighs are commonly affected. Lifting both arms above your head can be painful and difficult. The pain and stiffness are often worse in mornings. Other symptoms include a general feeling of being unwell and fatigue. It mainly affects people over the age of 70.

Some people who have polymyalgia rheumatica develop a condition called Giant Cell Arteritis (GCA). This affects the blood vessels in the head and can lead to symptoms of pain and tenderness around the side of the head. Giant cell arteritis can also cause pain in the tongue or jaw when chewing, and in rare cases problems with vision or even loss of vision. If you get any of these symptoms, it's important to see a doctor urgently. If left untreated, giant cell arteritis can lead to permanent damage to eyesight, even blindness. Both polymyalgia rheumatica and giant cell arteritis can be treated effectively with steroids, normally tablets. See Chapter 11 for more about Polymyalgia Rheumatica.

Secondary arthritis

In secondary arthritis, something identifiable triggers the degradation of the cartilage. In other words, the arthritis follows the injury. This type of arthritis is seen in people who have suffered a severe trauma or repetitive microtrauma to a joint. They may be obese or over-exert themselves (such as running a marathon without proper training). They may have abnormal body biomechanics, a term that refers to how the skeletal structures, including the bones, muscles, tendons, ligaments, and joints, function together -- meaning how they move through space under the influence of gravity.

People with a history of severe joint trauma, such as a broken bone or a torn knee ligament, may have suffered cartilage damage at the time of injury. This damage initiates a process of degeneration that can cause further cartilage damage and erosion. People who suffer repetitive microtrauma, such as a runner who wears improper footwear, may experience continual microtrauma to the joint cartilage.

Juvenile idiopathic arthritis (JIA)

If someone is diagnosed with inflammatory arthritis before their sixteenth birthday, it's called juvenile idiopathic arthritis, or JIA. There are different types of JIA. They are auto-immune conditions, and the immune system can cause pain and swelling in joints. The earlier someone is diagnosed with JIA, the better. This is so that effective treatment can be started and limit any damage to the body. See Chapter 12 for more about JIA.

General advice concerning arthritis

It's common to have aches and pains in your muscles and joints from time to time. This may especially be true if you take part in unusual or strenuous physical activities.

So, how can you tell the difference between the early signs of arthritis and normal pain and stiffness? And, how do you know when you should see a doctor about your symptoms? If you have swelling or stiffness that you can't explain and that won't go away in a few days, or if it becomes painful to touch your joints, you should see a doctor. The earlier you get a diagnosis and start the right type of treatment, the better the outcome will be. Here are some other things to think about that might help you decide whether you need to see a doctor:

Persistence of symptoms
- How and when did the pain start?
- If the pain came on after unusual exercise or activity you may have just overdone it a bit, and the pain should ease within a few days.
- See a doctor if the pain isn't linked to an injury or if the pain won't go away.

Swelling of joints
- If a joint becomes swollen, and isn't linked to an injury, you should see a doctor.
- This is especially important if you're also unwell or have a fever, or if the joint is red and warm.

Effects on your daily life
- See a doctor or other relevant healthcare professional if you're unable to do everyday tasks due to joint or muscle pain.
- If you've lifted something heavy and hurt your back, for example, take some painkillers, apply some heat and try to stay active. If the pain doesn't ease after a couple of weeks or so, see a doctor.

It's important to see a doctor if you get any new symptoms or if you have any trouble with drugs you're taking. If you have an appointment with a doctor, to help make sure you get the most out of it, you could take a list of questions with you and tick them off as they are discussed.

You could also keep a symptoms diary with details of how you're feeling in between appointments. Some people find that taking a friend or relative with them to an appointment can provide support and ensure that all important points are discussed.

Other conditions that have similar symptoms to arthritis
There are a number of other conditions that can cause pain and possibly swelling in and around joints.

Back pain

Back pain is a common problem that affects many of us. It's usually caused by a simple muscle or ligament strain and not usually by a serious problem. There might not even be a specific cause. Back pain will usually clear away in a couple of weeks. Remaining active while taking painkillers is often the best thing you can do.

Tendinopathy

Tendinopathy is a condition in which tendons, the strong cords that attach muscles to bones, are painful. The affected part of the body may be hot, swollen and red. This can make moving that part of the body difficult. You might also feel a grating sensation. This can be caused by over-use of that part of the body. Stopping or altering the activity that caused the problem may be the first step to recovery. Remaining generally active and taking painkillers can also help.

Applying an ice pack, such as a bag of frozen peas wrapped in a tea towel, can also reduce pain and swelling.

How can I help myself if I have arthritis?

As well as medical treatments, there are many things you can do to help yourself manage your arthritis. You might not always feel like exercising if you have arthritis. And you might be worried that exercising will make your pain or your condition worse. However, exercise can make symptoms such as pain and swelling better.

There are several reasons why this is the case:

- Your muscles will become stronger. This will provide better support to the joint.

18

- Your joints will become supple and less likely to become stiff.

- Your joints will be able to maintain their range of movement.

- Exercise improves your overall health and fitness and can help you maintain a healthy weight.

- Exercise leads to the release of chemicals in the body called endorphins. These are painkillers produced naturally by the body. Releasing them into the blood through exercise can make you feel good.

- Exercising regularly can help you get good sleep, which can help the body repair itself.

Type of exercise

People usually find that low-impact exercise is best. Swimming, cycling, brisk walking, yoga, Tai Chi, and Pilates are all examples of exercises that have helped people with arthritis. It's good to find something you enjoy so that you keep doing it.

You may feel some discomfort and sometimes pain when you exercise. This feeling is normal and should calm down a few minutes after you finish. It's not a sign that you are hurting yourself. Exercise will help reduce pain and can help you manage your arthritis better.

While you can push yourself and do strenuous exercise, it's important not to overdo it. If you are in pain that you can't cope with during or after your activity, you will need to see a doctor. The key is to start off gently and to gradually increase the amount you do.

Regular exercise is also an important part of maintaining a healthy weight. This will improve your symptoms as it will take pressure off joints. Being overweight can make someone more likely to have inflammation in their body. The best way to lose weight is to have a healthy, low-fat, low-sugar and balanced diet. Make sure you have plenty of fresh fruit and vegetables, drink plenty of water, and exercise regularly. If you burn off more calories than you consume on a daily basis, you will lose weight. If you are ever struggling and need support or motivation to keep active, see a GP or physiotherapist.

If you can afford it, another option would be to have regular sessions with a personal fitness trainer at a gym. If you are able to find someone who is trained to personal trainer level two or above, they will be able to give you advice on the best exercises for you and can monitor your progress. Make sure you tell them about your condition. See Chapter 13

Understanding your condition

Having a good understanding of your condition will help you know about your treatment options and why exercise and other self-management methods are important. It will also mean you're in a good position to get the most out of your appointments with healthcare professionals.

If you're ever struggling with any aspects of managing your arthritis, or notice new symptoms, you should see a GP. They could also refer you to another relevant healthcare professional. This could include a physiotherapist, who is trained to help you with exercise and help you maintain movement and function of any part of your body affected by arthritis.

Alternatively, you might benefit from seeing an occupational therapist. These are professionals who could help you overcome the difficulties that your condition might cause, by providing practical solutions. You can be referred to physiotherapists and occupational therapists on the NHS through your GP. If you are struggling with every-day tasks at home, you may be able to get access to an occupational therapist through your local social services department.

****

Chapter 2

Osteoarthritis

OSTEOARTHRITIS

NORMAL KNEE JOINT   OSTEOARTHRITIS

Osteoarthritis (OA) sometimes called degenerative joint disease is the most common chronic condition of the joints, affecting approximately 9.7 million people in the UK. Osteoarthritis can affect any of the joints, but occurs most often in the knees, hips, lower back and neck, small joints of the fingers and the bases of the thumb and big toe.

In healthy joints, a firm, smooth material, the cartilage covers the end of each bone. Cartilage provides a smooth, gliding surface for joint motion and acts as a cushion between the bones. In Osteoarthritis, the cartilage breaks down, causing pain, swelling and problems moving the joint. As OA worsens over time, bones may break down and develop growths called spurs. Bits of bone or cartilage may chip off and float around in the joint. In the body, an inflammatory process occurs and cytokines (proteins) and enzymes develop that further damage the cartilage. In the final stages of OA, the cartilage wears away and bone rubs against bone leading to joint damage and more pain. All in all, a painful and degenerative process.

Who's Affected?

Although it occurs in people of all ages, osteoarthritis is most common in people over the age of 65 and also women and people with a family history of the condition. Common risk factors include increasing age, obesity, previous joint injury, overuse of the joint, weak thigh muscles, and genes. It is a fact that:

- One in two adults will develop symptoms of knee OA during their lives.
- One in four adults will develop symptoms of hip OA by age 85.
- One in 12 people 60 years or older have hand OA.

Symptoms of osteoarthritis vary, depending on which joints are affected and how severely they are affected. However, the most common symptoms are pain and stiffness, particularly first thing in the morning or after resting. Affected joints may get swollen, especially after extended activity. These symptoms tend to build over time rather than show up suddenly. Some of the common symptoms include:

- Sore or stiff joints – particularly the hips, knees, and lower back – after inactivity or overuse.
- Limited range of motion or stiffness that goes away after movement
- Clicking or cracking sound when a joint bends
- Mild swelling around a joint
- Pain that is worse after activity or toward the end of the day

OA may affect different parts of the body in the following ways:

- **Hips.** Pain is felt in the groin area or buttocks and sometimes on the inside of the knee or thigh.
- **Knees.** A "grating" or "scraping" sensation occurs when moving the knee.
- **Fingers.** Bony growths (spurs) at the edge of joints can cause fingers to become swollen, tender and red. There may be pain at the base of the thumb.
- **Feet.** Pain and tenderness is felt in the large joint at the base of the big toe. There may be swelling in ankles or toes.

OA pain, swelling or stiffness may make it difficult to perform ordinary tasks at work or at home. Simple acts such as making the bed, opening boxes, grasping something such as a computer mouse or driving a car can become nearly impossible. When the lower body joints are affected, activities such as walking, climbing stairs and lifting objects may become difficult.

Many people believe that the effects of osteoarthritis are inevitable, so they don't do anything to manage it. OA symptoms can hinder work, social life and family life if steps are not taken to prevent joint damage, manage pain and increase flexibility.

How OA May Affect Overall Health

The pain, reduced mobility, side effects from medication and other factors associated with osteoarthritis can lead to negative health effects not directly related to the joint disease.

Diabetes and Heart Disease

Knee or hip pain may lead to a sedentary lifestyle that promotes weight gain and possible obesity. Being overweight or obese can lead to the development of diabetes, heart disease and high blood pressure.

Falls

People with osteoarthritis experience as much as 30 percent more falls and have a 20 percent greater risk of fracture than those without OA. People with OA have risk factors such as decreased function, muscle weakness and impaired balance that make them more likely to fall. Side effects from medications used for pain relief can also contribute to falls. Narcotic pain relievers can cause people to feel dizzy and unbalanced

Initial diagnosis of osteoarthritis

When first diagnosing osteoarthritis, a doctor will collect information from the patient on personal and family medical history and then perform a physical examination and order diagnostic tests. The information needed to help diagnose osteoarthritis includes:

- The patients description of the symptoms and details about when and how the pain or other symptoms began
- Details about other medical problems that exist
- Location of the pain, stiffness or other symptoms
- How the symptoms affect daily activities
- A list of current medications taken by the patient

During the exam, the doctor will examine the joints and test their range of motion (how well each joint moves through its full range). The doctor will be looking for areas that are tender, painful or swollen as well as signs of joint damage. They will examine the position and alignment of the neck and spine.

Diagnostic Tests

A diagnosis of osteoarthritis may be suspected after a medical history and physical examination is done. Blood tests are usually not helpful in making a diagnosis. However, the following tests may help confirm it:

- **Joint aspiration.** The doctor will numb the affected area and insert a needle into the joint to withdraw fluid. The fluid will be examined for evidence of crystals or joint deterioration. This test can help rule out other medical conditions or other forms of arthritis.
- **X-ray.** X-rays can show damage and other changes related to osteoarthritis to confirm the diagnosis.

- **MRI.** Magnetic resonance imaging (MRI) does not use radiation. It is more expensive than X-rays, but will provide a view that offers better images of cartilage and other structures to detect early abnormalities typical of osteoarthritis.

Osteoarthritis Treatment

As we have discussed, osteoarthritis is a chronic long-term disease. There is no absolute cure, but, very importantly, treatments are available to manage symptoms. Long-term management of the disease will include several factors:

- Managing symptoms, such as pain, stiffness and swelling
- Improving joint mobility and flexibility
- Maintaining a healthy weight
- Getting enough exercise

Physical Activity

One of the most beneficial ways to manage OA is to get moving. While it may be hard to think of exercise when the joints hurt, moving is considered an important part of the treatment plan. Studies show that simple activities like walking around the block or taking a fun, easy exercise class can reduce pain and help maintain (or attain) a healthy weight.

Strengthening exercises build muscles around OA-affected joints, easing the burden on those joints and reducing pain. Range-of-motion exercise helps maintain and improve joint flexibility and reduce stiffness. Aerobic exercise helps to improve stamina and energy levels and also help to reduce excess weight.

See the useful addresses and websites at the end of this chapter to get further advice about appropriate exercises. Also, see Chapter 13 for more information on exercises.

Weight Management

Excess weight adds additional stress to weight-bearing joints, such as the hips, knees, feet and back. Losing weight can help people with OA reduce pain and limit further joint damage. The basic rule for losing weight is to eat fewer calories and increase physical activity. The importance of diet is covered in chapter 13.

Stretching

Slow, gentle stretching of joints may improve flexibility, lessen stiffness and reduce pain. Exercises such as yoga and tai chi are great ways to manage stiffness.

Pain and Anti-inflammatory Medications

Medicines for osteoarthritis are available as pills, syrups, creams or lotions, or they are injected into a joint. They include:

- **Analgesics.** These are pain relievers and include acetaminophen, opioids (narcotics) and an atypical opioid called tramadol. They are available over-the-counter or by prescription.
- **Nonsteroidal anti-inflammatory drugs (NSAIDs).**
- These are the most commonly used drugs to ease inflammation and related pain. NSAIDs include aspirin, ibuprofen, naproxen. They are available over-the-counter or by prescription.

- **Corticosteroids.** Corticosteroids are powerful anti-inflammatory medicines. They are taken by mouth or injected directly into a joint.
- **Hyaluronic acid.** Hyaluronic acid occurs naturally in joint fluid, acting as a shock absorber and lubricant. However, the acid appears to break down in people with osteoarthritis.

Opioids

Opioids, such as codeine, are another type of painkiller that may ease your pain if paracetamol does not work. Opioids can help relieve severe pain, but can also cause side effects such as drowsiness, nausea and constipation. Codeine is found in combination with paracetamol in common preparations such as co-codamol.

Other opioids that may be prescribed for osteoarthritis include tramadol (brand names include Zamadol and Zydol), and dihydrocodeine (brand name DF 118 Forte). Both come in tablet form and as an injection.

Tramadol isn't suitable if you have uncontrolled epilepsy, and dihydrocodeine isn't recommended for patients with chronic obstructive pulmonary disease (COPD). If you need to take an opioid regularly, your GP may prescribe a laxative to take alongside it to prevent constipation.

Capsaicin cream

Your GP may prescribe capsaicin cream if you have osteoarthritis in your hands or knees and topical NSAIDs haven't been effective in easing your pain. Capsaicin cream works by blocking the nerves that send pain messages in the treated area. You may have to use it for a while before it has an effect. You should experience some pain relief within the first 2 weeks of using the cream, but it may take up to a month for the treatment to be fully effective.

Apply a pea-sized amount of capsaicin cream to your affected joints up to 4 times a day, but not more often than every 4 hours. Don't use capsaicin cream on broken or inflamed skin and always wash your hands after applying it.

Be careful not to get any capsaicin cream on delicate areas, such as your eyes, mouth, nose and genitals. Capsaicin is made from chillies, so if you get it on sensitive areas of your body, it's likely to be very painful for a few hours. However, it won't cause any damage.

You may notice a burning sensation on your skin after applying capsaicin cream. This is nothing to worry about, and the more you use it, the less it should happen. But avoid using too much cream or having a hot bath or shower before or after applying it, because it can make the burning sensation worse.

Steroid injections
Steroids are a type of medication that contain man made versions of the hormone cortisol, and are sometimes used to treat particularly painful musculoskeletal problems. Some people with osteoarthritis may be offered steroid injections when other treatments haven't worked. The injection will be made directly into the affected area. You may be given a local anaesthetic first to numb the area and reduce the pain.

Steroid injections are only likely to provide short-term relief. If steroid injections are helping, you may be offered up to 3 injections in the same area, with at least a 3 to 6 month gap between them.

PRP injections

Platelet rich plasma (PRP) is a newer treatment that may be offered to treat osteoarthritis. PRP is blood plasma containing concentrated platelets that your body uses to repair damaged tissue. Injections of PRP have been shown to speed up the healing process in some people but their long-term effectiveness is not yet known.

The surgeon will take a blood sample from you and place it in a machine. This separates the healing platelets so they can be taken from the blood sample and injected into the affected joints. The procedure usually takes about 15 minutes.

Supportive treatments

In addition to lifestyle changes and medication, you may also benefit from a number of supportive treatments that can help reduce your pain and make everyday tasks easier.

Transcutaneous electrical nerve stimulation (TENS)

Transcutaneous electrical nerve stimulation (TENS) uses a machine that sends electrical impulses through sticky patches, called electrodes, attached to the skin. This may help ease the pain caused by your osteoarthritis by numbing the nerve endings in your spinal cord which control pain. Treatment with TENS is usually arranged by a physiotherapist, who can advise on the strength of the pulses and how long your treatment should last.

Hot or cold packs

Applying hot or cold packs (sometimes called thermotherapy or cryotherapy) to the joints can relieve the pain and symptoms of osteoarthritis in some people. A hot-water bottle filled with either hot or cold water and applied to the affected area can be very effective in reducing pain. Special hot and cold packs that can either be cooled in the freezer or heated in a microwave are also available, and work in a similar way.

Manual therapy

Not using your joints can cause your muscles to waste and may increase stiffness caused by osteoarthritis. Manual therapy is a treatment provided by a physiotherapist. It uses stretching techniques to keep your joints supple and flexible.

Physical and Occupational Therapy

Physical and occupational therapists can provide a range of treatment options for pain management including:

- Ways to properly use joints
- Heat and cold therapies
- Range of motion and flexibility exercises
- Assistive devices

Assistive Devices

Assistive devices can help with function and mobility. These include items, such as scooters, canes, walkers, splints, shoe orthotics or helpful tools, such as jar openers, long-handled shoe horns or steering wheel grips. Many devices can be found at pharmacies and medical supply stores. But some items, such as custom knee braces and shoe wedges are prescribed by a doctor and are typically fitted by a physical or occupational therapist.

Natural and Alternative Therapies

Many people with OA use natural or alternative therapies to address symptoms and improve their overall well-being. These include nutritional supplements, acupuncture or acupressure, massage, relaxation techniques and hydrotherapy, among others. Many of these alternative medicines and therapies are perfectly legitimate and do indeed help sufferers. However, sad to say that the arthritis industry attracts many charlatans who offer all sorts of pills and potions to cure arthritis or at least minimise the pain. Be very careful before parting with any money. Do your research on products and see what others have to say about them.

Surgery

Joint surgery can repair or replace severely damaged joints, especially hips or knees. A doctor will refer an eligible patient to an orthopaedic surgeon to perform the procedure.

Positive Attitude

Many studies have demonstrated that a positive outlook can boost the immune system and increase a person's ability to handle pain. This is difficult, and also easy to say, but by getting in touch with one of the organisations listed below, you can at least improve the state of your mind by sharing experiences.

****

Organisations providing useful advice and support

With the right support, you can lead a healthy, active life with osteoarthritis. Osteoarthritis doesn't necessarily get worse and doesn't always lead to disability. Many people find it helpful to talk to other people who are in a similar position to them. You may find support from a group or by talking individually to someone who has osteoarthrits. Patient organisations have local groups where you can meet other people with the same

Versus Arthritis (formerly Arthritis Care and Arthritis Research UK)

Copeman House, St Mary's Court

St Mary's Gate

Chesterfield S41 7TD

Phone: 0300 790 0400

versusarthritis.org.

Email: enquiries@versusarthritis.org

Versus Arthritis was formed in 2018 following a merger of Arthritis Care and Arthritis Research UK. They campaign to challenge the misconceptions around arthritis and to ensure it is recognised as priority in the UK. They offer very useful support and guidance including an online forum. Versus Arthritis offers support and Guidance in the whole of the UK, including Scotland Wales and Northern Ireland.

Entitlement to benefits and other support

If you have severe osteoarthritis and are still working, your symptoms may interfere with your working life and may affect your ability to do your job. Versus Arthritis has useful advice on how you can make simple adjustments at work to make it easier to do your job. If you have to stop work or work part time because of your arthritis, you may find it hard to cope financially. You may be entitled to one or more of the following types of financial support:

- if you have a job but can't work because of your illness, you are entitled to Statutory Sick Pay from your employer
- if you do not have a job and cannot work because of your illness, you may be entitled to Employment and Support Allowance
- if you are aged 64 or under and need help with personal care or have walking difficulties, you may be eligible for the Personal Independence Payment
- if you are aged 65 or over, you may be able to get Attendance Allowance
- if you are caring for someone with rheumatoid arthritis, you may be entitled to Carer's Allowance

You may be eligible for other benefits if you have children living at home or if you have a low household income. For more information go to:

GOV.UK: benefits

The NHS has a very useful website:

www.nhs.uk/conditions/social-care-and-support-guide: This site covers all topics relating to different forms of arthritis and what care and support can be accessed including therapists and local support groups. Another extremely useful website is that of the Money Advice Service:

www.moneyadviceservice.org.uk/en/articles/how-to-sort-out-your-money-if-you-become-ill-or-disabled.

This site offers comprehensive coverage of help and support when a person becomes ill or disabled.

****

Chapter 3

Rheumatoid Arthritis

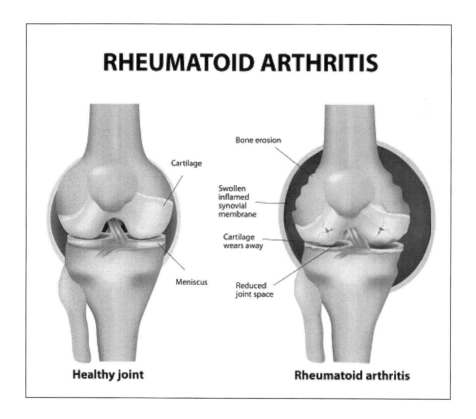

Rheumatoid arthritis **(RA)** is a long-term autoimmune disorder that primarily affects joints. It typically results in warm, swollen, and painful joints. Pain and stiffness often worsen following rest. Most commonly, the wrist and hands are involved, with the same joints typically involved on both sides of the body. The disease may also affect other parts of the body. This may result in a low red blood cell count, inflammation around the lungs, and inflammation around the heart. Fever and low energy may also be present. Often, symptoms come on gradually over weeks to months.

While the cause of rheumatoid arthritis is not clear, it is believed to involve a combination of genetic and environmental factors. The underlying mechanism involves the body's immune system attacking the joints. This results in inflammation and thickening of the joint capsule. It also affects the underlying bone and cartilage. The diagnosis (see below) is made mostly on the basis of a person's signs and symptoms. X-rays and laboratory testing may support a diagnosis or exclude other diseases with similar symptoms. Other diseases that may present similarly include psoriatic arthritis, and fibromyalgia among others.

Recent study-Infrared test can diagnose rheumatoid arthritis in minutes
Infrared scans could detect arthritis within two minutes and give thousands of patients quicker access to treatment before their symptoms set in, research has suggested.

A pilot study found that infrared scanners could accurately identify rheumatoid arthritis, a condition that affects about half a million people in the UK. At present, diagnosis involves examination by a hospital specialist followed by blood tests and costly x-rays, MRI or ultrasound scans. Hamid Dehghani, who led the University of Birmingham study, said that he expected table-top infrared scanners to give cheap and quick diagnoses at rheumatology clinics and GP surgeries within two to five years.

Unlike the more common osteoarthritis, which is caused when the cartilage in joints wears down over time, rheumatoid arthritis develops when the immune system attacks the joints, causing pain and swelling. Treatments are available but to be effective they must be delivered as soon as possible after the onset of the disease, often before any signs of arthritis are visible to the eye. In the study, researchers scanned the fingers of 21 patients with diagnosed rheumatoid arthritis using an infrared scanner and compared the results with those obtained by ultrasound and examination by a specialist. They found that the scanner detected signs of the disease with 88 per cent accuracy. It works by beaming infrared light through each finger and showing the results on a 3D digital image of the hand. Measuring the spectrum of light that has travelled through each finger allows scientists to identify levels of blood, water and oxygen, which in turn tell them whether there is inflammation in the joints.

Dr Dehghani said that the results, published in the *Journal of Biomedical Optics*, showed that the technology could be used to monitor progression of the disease and effectiveness of treatments, as well as being a diagnostic tool. "This could be a quick way to diagnose rheumatoid arthritis in no more than two to three minutes", he said. "In the future we are hopeful GPs will not have to send a patient to hospital to be examined by a specialist and scanned with expensive equipment. We envisage they will be able to use a shoe-box-sized device in their office. In rheumatology departments it will be a lot quicker and easier for a non-specialist to use an infrared scanner than ultrasound".

Diagnosing Rheumatoid Arthritis

Diagnosing rheumatoid arthritis quickly is important because early treatment can help stop the condition getting worse and reduce the risk of further problems such as joint damage.

Seeing your GP

Your GP will carry out a physical examination, checking your joints for any swelling and to assess how easily they move. They will also ask you about your symptoms. It's important to tell your GP about all your symptoms, not just ones you think are important, as this will help them make the correct diagnosis.

If your GP thinks you have rheumatoid arthritis, they'll refer you to a specialist (rheumatologist).

Blood tests

Your GP may arrange blood tests to help confirm the diagnosis. No blood test can definitively prove or rule out a diagnosis of rheumatoid arthritis, but a number of tests can show possible indications of the condition. Some of the main tests used include:

- erythrocyte sedimentation rate (ESR)
- C-reactive protein (CRP)
- full blood count

The full blood count measures your red cells to rule out anaemia. Anaemia means the blood is unable to carry enough oxygen because of a lack of blood cells.

Anaemia is common in people with rheumatoid arthritis, although having anaemia doesn't prove you have rheumatoid arthritis.

Rheumatoid factor and anti-CCP antibodies

As we have stated, specific blood tests can help diagnose rheumatoid arthritis, but aren't accurate in everyone. About half of all people with rheumatoid arthritis have a positive rheumatoid factor present in their blood when the disease starts, but about 1 in 20 people without rheumatoid arthritis also test positive.

An antibody test known as anti-cyclic citrullinated peptide (anti-CCP) is available. People who test positive for anti-CCP are very likely to develop rheumatoid arthritis, but not everybody found to have rheumatoid arthritis has this antibody. Those who test positive for both rheumatoid factor and anti-CCP may be more likely to have severe rheumatoid arthritis requiring higher levels of treatment.

Joint imaging

A number of different scans may also be carried out to check for joint inflammation and damage. These can help tell the difference between different types of arthritis and can be used to monitor how your condition is progressing over time. Scans that may be carried out to diagnose and monitor rheumatoid arthritis include:

- X-rays (where radiation is passed through your body to examine your bones and joints)
- MRI scans (where strong magnetic fields and radio waves are used to produce detailed images of your joints)

Assessing your physical ability

If you have been diagnosed with rheumatoid arthritis, your specialist will carry out an assessment to see how well you're coping with everyday tasks. You may be asked to fill in a questionnaire on how well you can do things like dress, walk and eat, and how good your grip strength is. This assessment may be repeated later on after your treatment to see if you have made any improvements.

Treatments for Rheumatoid Arthritis

Treatment for rheumatoid arthritis can help reduce inflammation in the joints, relieve pain, prevent or slow joint damage, reduce disability and enable you to live as active a life as possible. The goals of treatment are to reduce pain, decrease inflammation, and improve a person's overall functioning.

Although most alternative medicine treatments are not supported by evidence it is of course up to the individual whether or not they pursue them.

It is important to note that although there's no cure for rheumatoid arthritis, early treatment and support (including lifestyle changes, medication, supportive treatments and surgery) can reduce the risk of joint damage and limit the impact of the condition.

Your treatment will usually involve care from your GP and a number of different specialists. The National Institute for Health and Care Excellence (NICE) has produced guidance on the management of rheumatoid arthritis in adults.

There are a number of medications available that can be used to help stop rheumatoid arthritis getting worse and reduce your risk of further problems. These are often divided into 2 types of medication: disease-modifying anti-rheumatic drugs (DMARDs) and biological treatments.

Disease-modifying anti-rheumatic drugs (DMARDs)

If you have been diagnosed with rheumatoid arthritis, you'll normally be offered a combination of DMARD tablets as part of your initial treatment. These medications are particularly effective at easing symptoms of the condition and slowing down its progression. DMARDs work by blocking the effects of the chemicals released when the immune system attacks the joints, which could otherwise cause further damage to nearby bones, tendons, ligaments and cartilage. There are many different DMARDs that can be used, including:

- methotrexate
- leflunomide
- hydroxychloroquine
- sulfasalazine

Methotrexate is normally the first medicine given for rheumatoid arthritis, often alongside another DMARD and a short-course of corticosteroids to relieve any pain. It may also be combined with the biological treatments mentioned below. Common side effects of methotrexate include:

- feeling sick
- loss of appetite
- a sore mouth
- diarrhoea
- headaches
- hair loss

The medication can also sometimes have an effect on your blood count and your liver, so you'll have regular blood tests to monitor this.

Less commonly, methotrexate can affect the lungs, so you'll usually have a chest X-ray and possibly breathing tests when you start taking it to provide a comparison if you develop shortness of breath or a persistent dry cough while taking it. But most people tolerate methotrexate well.

It can take a few months to notice a DMARD working. It's important to keep taking the medication, even if you don't notice it working at first. You may have to try 2 or 3 types of DMARD before you find the one that's most suitable for you. Once you and your doctor work out the most suitable DMARD, you'll usually have to take the medicine in the long term.

Biological treatments
Biological treatments are a newer form of treatment for rheumatoid arthritis. They include:

- etanercept
- infliximab
- adalimumab

- certolizumab
- golimumab
- rituximab
- abatacept
- tocilizumab
- sarilumab

They're usually taken in combination with methotrexate or another DMARD, and are normally only used if these medications alone haven't been effective.

Biological medications are given by injection. They work by stopping particular chemicals in the blood from activating your immune system to attack your joints. It is important to understand the side effects of these treatments, which can be obtained from the NHS website of the NICE (National Association for Clinical Excellence) website

Side effects from biological treatments are usually mild and include:

- skin reactions at the site of the injections
- infections
- feeling sick
- a high temperature (fever)
- headaches

Some people may also be at risk of getting more serious problems, including the reactivation of infections such as Tuberculosis (TB) if they have had them in the past.

Complications of rheumatoid arthritis

Having rheumatoid arthritis can put you at a higher risk of developing other conditions:

- Carpal tunnel syndrome - this is a common condition in people with rheumatoid arthritis. Carpal tunnel syndrome is when there is too much pressure on the nerve in the wrist. It can cause aching, numbness and tingling in your thumb, fingers and part of the hand.

- Inflammation-because rheumatoid arthritis is an inflammatory condition, it can sometimes cause inflammation to develop in other parts of your body, such as your lungs, heart, blood vessels or eyes.

- Tendon rupture - tendons are pieces of flexible tissue that attach muscle to bone. Rheumatoid arthritis can cause your tendons to be become inflamed, which in severe cases can cause them to rupture. This most commonly affects the tendons on the backs of the fingers.

- Cervical myelopathy - if you have had rheumatoid arthritis for some time, you are at increased risk of developing cervical myelopathy and you may need special assessment of your neck before any operation where you are put to sleep. This condition is caused by dislocation of joints at the top of the spine, which put pressure on the spinal cord. Although relatively uncommon, it is a serious condition that can greatly affect your mobility.

- Vasculitis - this is a rare condition that causes inflammation of the blood vessels. It can lead to the thickening, weakening, narrowing and scarring of blood vessel walls. In serious cases, it can affect blood flow to your body's organs and tissues.

Living with rheumatoid arthritis

Rheumatoid arthritis can be life changing. You may need long-term treatment to control your symptoms and reduce joint damage. Depending on how much pain and stiffness you feel and how much joint damage you have, you may have to adapt the way you do simple daily tasks. They can become difficult or take a little longer to complete.

Self-care

Self-care is an integral part of daily life. It involves taking responsibility for your own health and wellbeing with support from the people involved in your care. Self care includes the things you do each day to stay fit, maintain good physical and mental health, prevent illness or accidents, and effectively deal with minor ailments and long-term conditions. People living with long-term conditions can benefit enormously if they receive support for self-care. They can live longer, have less pain, anxiety, depression and fatigue, have a better quality of life and are more active and independent.

Medication

It is important to take your medication as prescribed, even if you start to feel better. Continuous medication can help prevent flare-ups. If you have any questions or concerns about the medication you are taking or side effects, talk to your healthcare team. It may also be useful to read the information leaflet that comes with the medication about possible interactions with other drugs or supplements. Check with your healthcare team before taking any over-the-counter remedies, such as painkillers, or any nutritional supplements. These can sometimes interfere with your medication.

Regular reviews
Because rheumatoid arthritis is a long-term condition, you will be in contact with your healthcare team regularly. The more the team knows, the more they can help you, so discuss your symptoms or any concerns with them.

Keeping well
Everyone with a long-term condition, such as rheumatoid arthritis, is encouraged to get a yearly flu jab each autumn to protect against flu. They are also recommended to get an anti-pneumoccocal vaccination. This is a one-off injection that protects against a serious chest infection called pneumococcal pneumonia.

Get plenty of rest during a flare-up as this is when your joints can be particularly painful and inflamed. Putting further strain on very swollen and painful joints can often make pain and inflammation worse.

Healthy eating and exercise
Regular exercise and a healthy diet are recommended for everyone, not just people with rheumatoid arthritis. They can help prevent many conditions, including heart disease and many forms of cancer.

Exercising regularly can help relieve stress and reduce fatigue. A gentle form of exercise that does not put too much strain on your joints is best. Swimming, for example, helps exercise your muscles but puts very little strain on your joints because the water supports your weight. See chapter 13 for more on diet and exercise.

Starting and raising a family

If you're taking medicines for rheumatoid arthritis, let your healthcare team know if you want to start a family or you're worried about becoming pregnant while on medication. Some medications, such as methotrexate, leflunomide and biological treatments, shouldn't be taken by men or women while they're trying for a baby.

The doctors and nurses will work with you to ensure your rheumatoid arthritis is controlled while you're trying to get pregnant. Babies and young children are physically and mentally demanding for any parent, but particularly so if you have rheumatoid arthritis.

If you're struggling to cope, it may help to talk to other people in the same situation as you. You may also be able to get additional support from your health visitor or occupational therapist to help you manage your young family.

In addition, The National Rheumatoid Arthritis Society offers invaluable advice and support for would be parents (see overleaf).

****

Organisations providing useful advice and support

National Rheumatoid Arthritis Society
Freephone Helpline 0800 298 7650
email helpline@nras.org.uk
www.nras.org.uk

This is the main organisation providing advice and support for those suffering from Rheumatoid arthritis. If you are newly diagnosed with Rheumatoid Arthritis (RA), you suspect you have RA, or looking for information about treatments, exercise or lifestyle then the National Rheumatoid Arthritis Society will be an invaluable resource.

****

Chapter 4

Ankylosing Spondylitis and Enteropathic Arthritis

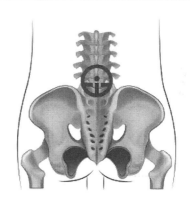

ANKYLOSING SPONDYLITIS

Ankylosing spondylitis

Ankylosing spondylitis is a chronic, long-term disease and can affect people over many years. It is a type of arthritis that mainly affects the joints in your spine. It causes pain and stiffness in the lower back. Although, generally, you can develop ankylosing spondylitis at any age, it usually starts in the late teens or early twenties. It is more prevalent amongst men than women. The symptoms can come and go, and many people have periods of feeling well for many months at a time. And for a lot of people, the symptoms will stay mild and won't cause any significant problems at all.

With ankylosing spondylitis, the joints in the spine become inflamed and worn down. As your body tries to repair the damage, it starts to produce new bone. In some people, if the disease progresses, this can eventually cause the bones of the spine to join together. Usually, it's the lower back and pelvis that are affected although other joints can be affected too, including the hips and the shoulders, and also the wall of your chest.

Ankylosing spondylitis belongs to a group of conditions called spondyloarthritis. You may sometimes hear ankylosing spondylitis referred to as 'axial spondyloarthritis', which means it affects your spine and central skeleton. Other types of spondyloarthritis affect your peripheral joints such as your knees and wrists.

Symptoms of ankylosing spondylitis

Symptoms of ankylosing spondylitis tend to develop slowly over several years. The symptoms may be very mild at first, and you may not know that you have the condition, but they might slowly get more noticeable over time and pain starts to set in. There may be times when the symptoms temporarily get worse followed by a remission. The main symptoms of ankylosing spondylitis are pain and stiffness in your lower back. The pain usually gets better when you move around. You might also feel pain in your buttocks and base of your thighs too.

Ankylosing spondylitis can also cause symptoms in other parts of your body. These symptoms may include pain in other joints such as your neck, shoulders, chest and hips, pain in areas of the body where tendons attach to a bone (this is called enthesitis and includes your elbows, knees and heels), and inflammation of your eye. Your eye may be red and painful, and you might become sensitive to bright lights. If you develop this, seek medical help straight away to prevent permanent damage. Finally, you might feel weak and frequently tired.

Carrying out a diagnosis of ankylosing spondylitis

In the initial diagnosis, your GP will ask about your symptoms and medical history, and will also want to do a physical examination. This will involve checking a range of movements, and also feeling your back for any tenderness in the joints. If your GP thinks your back pain could be due to ankylosing spondylitis, they will refer you to a rheumatologist to confirm the diagnosis. You will usually have several tests to help diagnose ankylosing spondylitis, including blood tests for proteins that can be a sign of inflammation in your body. and another blood test for the gene HLA-B27, which many people with ankylosing spondylitis have. Also it is usually necessary to have an X-ray of the bones and joints in your back and an MRI scan of your back.

Treatment of ankylosing spondylitis

As we have stated, ankylosing spondylitis is a long-term condition – it isn't something that can be absolutely cured. However, there's a lot you can do to help manage your condition, and treatments are available to ease any symptoms you have. This should help to reduce the impact the disease has on your everyday life.

Physiotherapy and exercise

Physiotherapy is an important part of treatment for ankylosing spondylitis. When you're diagnosed with the condition, your doctor will almost certainly suggest you see a physiotherapist, who will then put together an exercise programme tailored to your needs. The programme of exercises will be designed to help you to stay as flexible and mobile as possible. It should include some of the following.

- Exercises to help stretch and strengthen your back.
- Exercises to help maintain a good posture.
- Deep breathing exercises, to help expand your chest muscles.
- Exercises that extend your spine.
- Exercises that work the different sections of your spine and help to improve your range of movement in each area.
- Aerobic exercise (exercises that increase your heart rate and get you out of breath).
- Hydrotherapy – doing special exercises in a heated pool. This may help to manage your pain and improve how much you can move.

Medicines

Painkillers and anti-inflammatory medicines

In the first instance, you'll usually be offered treatment with non-steroidal anti-inflammatory drugs (NSAIDs). These help reduce pain and the stiffness in the joints. These medicines should help to slow down any worsening of your condition. However, It is very important that you take them regularly. If the particular medicine you're given doesn't help within a few weeks, your doctor may adjust your dose or try a different medicine.

If you take NSAIDs regularly, your doctor may suggest you take a medicine called a proton pump inhibitor as well. This will protect your stomach and reduce the risk of side-effects from NSAIDs. If you can't take NSAIDs for any reason or they're not helping enough, your doctor may suggest a different painkiller such as paracetamol or codeine. If you have a particularly painful and swollen joint, your doctor may suggest a steroid injection into the joint.

Corticosteroids

Corticosteroids have a powerful anti-inflammatory effect and can be taken as tablets or injections by people with AS. If a particular joint is inflamed, corticosteroids can be injected directly into the joint. You'll need to rest the joint for up to 48 hours after the injection. It's usually considered wise to have a corticosteroid injection up to three times in one year, with at least three months between injections in the same joint. This is because corticosteroids injections can cause a number of side effects, such as:

- infection in response to the injection
- the skin around the injection may change colour (depigmentation)
- the surrounding tissue may waste away
- a tendon near the joint may burst (rupture)

Corticosteroids may also calm down painful swollen joints when taken as tablets.

Disease-modifying anti-rheumatic drugs

Your GP might recommend treatment with a disease-modifying anti-rheumatic drug (DMARD). There are different types of

DMARD. Newer DMARDs include a group of medicines known as tumour necrosis factor (TNF) blockers, or biological DMARDs. They include the medicines etanercept, adalimumab and golimumab, certolizumab pegol and secukinumab. These drugs target your immune system to reduce inflammation. They might be recommended if your symptoms are severe and haven't been controlled by other treatments. These drugs are injected under the skin, which you can do yourself. Your doctor will monitor your response to these drugs closely and only continue with treatment if it's having a clear benefit.

NICE Guidelines

The National Institute for Health and Care Excellence (NICE) has produced guidance about the use of anti-TNF medication for AS. NICE states adalimumab, etanercept and golimumab may only be used if:

- your diagnosis of ankylosing spondylitis has been confirmed
- your level of pain is assessed twice (using a simple scale that you fill in) 12 weeks apart and confirms your condition has not improved
- your Bath Ankylosing Spondylitis Disease Activity Index (BASDAI) is tested twice, 12 weeks apart, and confirms your condition has not improved – BASDAI is a set of measures devised by experts to evaluate your condition by asking a number of questions about your symptoms
- treatment with two or more NSAIDs for four weeks at the highest possible dose has not controlled your symptoms

After 12 weeks of treatment with anti-TNF medication, your pain score and BASDAI will be tested again to see whether they've improved enough to make continuing treatment worthwhile. If they have, treatment will continue and you'll be tested every 12 weeks. If there's not enough improvement after 12 weeks, you'll be tested again at a later date or the treatment will be stopped.

Surgery

Most people with ankylosing spondylitis don't need surgery. But if one of your joints such as your hip or shoulder is severely affected, your doctor may suggest having it replaced. A small number of people with a fused and bent spine that's severely affecting their quality of life may have an operation to correct it.

Causes of ankylosing spondylitis

The causes of ankylosing spondylitis are not clear. However, It's known that there is a strong genetic link and the condition often runs in families. Having a gene called HLA-B27 makes it more likely to develop the condition, especially if you also have a close relative with the condition. There are also other genes involved, and environmental factors seem to trigger the disease in certain people.

Complications of ankylosing spondylitis

If you've had severe disease for a long time, you may be at greater risk of developing complications. These may include: spinal fractures – you're at greater risk of this if the bones in your spine have joined together (fused), Osteoporosis – this is when your bones become weak and brittle, which can make them more likely to break. Up to three in 10 people with ankylosing spondylitis are thought to develop osteoporosis, Heart problems – people with ankylosing spondylitis seem to be at greater risk of developing problems with their heart and circulation.

However, reassuringly, it is a fact that most people with ankylosing spondylitis don't develop severe disability or any other complications.

Living with ankylosing spondylitis

Like many such conditions, ankylosing spondylitis will affect people in different ways. It is a fact that most people will have very mild symptoms that cause few problems. However, some people may go on to have significant disability. When you're first diagnosed, your doctor should talk you through how to deal with any flare-ups. This might include who you can contact if you need help (for example, a rheumatology nurse). Dealing with flare-ups also includes stretches and exercises you can do, and information on how to manage pain and fatigue.

If you're having difficulties with everyday activities, your doctor may refer you to a specialist such as an occupational therapist for advice. They'll be able to advise you on any changes you can make or devices you may be able to use to make life easier. You might need to make changes to your work environment, especially if you have a physically demanding job, so you can do your job safely.

Enteropathic arthritis

Enteropathic arthritis is an inflammatory condition affecting the spine and other joints that commonly occurs in the inflammatory bowel diseases – Crohn's disease and ulcerative colitis. Inflammatory arthritis associated with other enteropathic diseases, such as like celiac disease and Whipple's disease, are not generally included in "enteropathic arthritis."

Enteropathic arthritis is classified as one of the spondyloarthropathies. Other spondyloarthropathies include ankylosing spondylitis, psoriatic arthritis, and reactive arthritis. "Enteropathy" refers to any disease related to the intestines.

Symptoms

Enteropathic arthritis may occur as axial arthritis, peripheral arthritis, or mixed. As axial arthritis, symptoms of back pain and stiffness resemble ankylosing spondylitis and may precede gastrointestinal symptoms. As peripheral arthritis, there is typically a pattern of pauciarticular (four or fewer joints involved) and asymmetric arthritis (affected joints are not on the same side of the body). The gastrointestinal problems can occur at the same time as arthritis or arthritis can occur before bowel disease.

Causes

Arthritis occurs in up to 20 percent of people who have inflammatory bowel disease, with higher prevalence among those with Crohn's disease compared to those with ulcerative colitis. In enteropathic arthritis, the arthritis symptoms can precede the gastrointestinal symptoms for a long period of time.

Until the gastrointestinal symptoms are apparent, the arthritis is often classified as Undifferentiated Spondyloarthritis. Most people with enteropathic arthritis, however, have already been diagnosed with one of the inflammatory bowel diseases.

**

Diagnosis

An open and honest discussion with your doctor about all of your symptoms is the place to start. Typically doctors do tests to look for:

- anemia
- elevated CRP and ESR indicative of inflammation
- lack of erosive changes on an x-ray of peripheral joints
- sacroiliac and spine x-rays that resemble ankylosing spondylitis

Treatment

Enteropathic arthritis is treated much the same as other spondyloarthropathies for joint symptoms. The problem is that both conditions must be dealt with—the arthritis as well as the bowel disease—but as NSAIDs may effectively treat arthritis, the drugs may make bowel disease worse.

TNF inhibitors, which include Remicade (infliximab), Humira (adalimumab) and Cimzia (certolizumab pegol) have been successfully used to treat inflammatory bowel disease. They are also effective for inflammatory arthritis.

****

Organisations providing useful advice and support

National Ankylosing Spondylitis Society

The National Ankylosing Spondylitis Society (NASS) is the only charity dedicated to transforming the lives of people with AS in the UK. They strive to raise awareness of AS, and provide life-changing support to anyone affected, including friends and family. They can be contacted at:

172 King Street,

Hammersmith,

London,

W6 0QU

Tel: 020 8741 1515

www.nass.co.uk

NHS website

www.nhs.uk/conditions/Ankylosing-spondylitis

The NHS information and support website offers very useful advice and guidance.

Below are websites for very useful online support group, which have a blog where you can contact other people with the condition.

www.dailystrength.org/group/ankylosing-spondylitis

ankylosingspondylitisnews.com

WebMD

www.webmd.com/arthritis/ankylosing-spondylitis-support

Chapter 5

Cervical Spondylitis

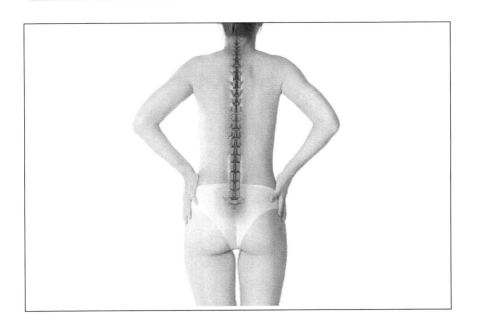

Cervical spondylosis

Cervical spondylosis is an age-related condition that affects the joints and discs in the cervical spine, which is in the neck. It is also commonly referred to as cervical osteoarthritis or neck arthritis. It develops from the wear and tear of cartilage and bones. While it's largely the result of age, it can be caused by other factors as well. Although some people who have it never experience symptoms, for others, it can cause chronic, severe pain and stiffness.

Causes of cervical spondylosis

The bones and protective cartilage in your neck are prone to wear and tear that can lead to cervical spondylosis. Possible causes of the condition include:

Bone spurs

These overgrowths of bone are the result of the body trying to grow extra bone to make the spine stronger. However, the extra bone can press on delicate areas of the spine, such as the spinal cord and nerves, resulting in pain.

Dehydrated spinal discs.

Spinal bones have discs between them, which are thick, pad like cushions that absorb the shock of lifting, twisting, and other activities. The gel-like material inside these discs can dry out over time. This causes bones (spinal vertebrae) to rub together more, which can be painful.

Herniated discs

Spinal discs can develop cracks, which allows leakage of the internal cushioning material. This material can press on the spinal cord and nerves, resulting in symptoms such as arm numbness as well as pain that radiates down an arm.

Injury

If you've had an injury to your neck (during a fall for example), this can accelerate the aging process.

**

Ligament stiffness
The tough cords that connect spinal bones to each other can become even stiffer over time, which affects neck movement and makes the neck feel tight.

Overuse
Some occupations or hobbies involve repetitive movements or heavy lifting (such as building work). This can put extra pressure on the spine, resulting in early wear and tear.

Risk factors for the condition
The greatest risk factor for cervical spondylosis is aging. Cervical spondylosis often develops as a result of changes in your neck joints as you age. Disc herniation, dehydration, and bone spurs are all results of aging. Factors other than aging can increase your risk of cervical spondylosis. These include:

neck injuries
Work-related activities that put extra strain on your neck from heavy lifting, holding your neck in an uncomfortable position for prolonged periods of time or repeating the same neck movements throughout the day (repetitive stress),genetic factors (family history of cervical spondylosis).

Smoking presents a risk, as does being overweight and inactive.

Symptoms of cervical spondylosis
Most people with cervical spondylosis don't have significant symptoms. If symptoms do occur, they can range from mild to severe and may develop gradually or occur suddenly. One

common symptom is pain around the shoulder blade. Some complain of pain along the arm and in the fingers. The pain might increase when:

- standing
- sitting
- sneezing
- coughing
- tilting your neck backward

Another common symptom is muscle weakness. Muscle weakness makes it hard to lift the arms or grasp objects firmly. Other common signs include:

- a stiff neck that becomes worse
- headaches that mostly occur in the back of the head
- tingling or numbness that mainly affects the shoulders and arms, although it can also occur in the legs

Symptoms that occur less frequently often include a loss of balance and a loss of bladder or bowel control. These symptoms warrant immediate medical attention.

When to see a doctor

If you have the sudden onset of numbness or tingling in the shoulder, arms, or legs, or if you lose bowel or bladder control, talk to your doctor and seek medical attention as soon as possible. Although the condition is often the result of aging, there are treatments available that can reduce pain and stiffness.

Testing for and diagnosing the condition

Making a diagnosis of cervical spondylosis involves ruling out other potential conditions, such as fibromyalgia (Chapter 6). Making a diagnosis also involves testing for movement and determining the affected nerves, bones, and muscles. Your doctor may treat your condition or refer you to an orthopaedic specialist, neurologist, or neurosurgeon for further testing.

Physical exam

Your doctor will start by asking you several questions regarding your symptoms. Then, they'll run through a set of tests. Typical exams include testing your reflexes, checking for muscle weakness or sensory deficits, and testing the range of motion of your neck. Your doctor might also want to watch how you walk. All of this helps your doctor determine if your nerves and spinal cord are under too much pressure. If your doctor suspects cervical spondylosis, they'll then order imaging tests and nerve function tests to confirm the diagnosis.

Imaging tests

X-rays can be used to check for bone spurs and other abnormalities. A CT scan can provide more detailed images of your neck. An MRI scan, which produces images using radio waves and a magnetic field, helps your doctor locate pinched nerves. In a myelogram, a dye injection is used to highlight certain areas of your spine. CT scans or X-rays are then used to provide more detailed images of these areas.

An electromyogram (EMG) is used to check that your nerves are functioning normally when sending signals to your muscles. This test measures your nerves' electrical activity. This is done by placing electrodes on your skin where the nerve is located.

Treating cervical spondylosis

Treatments for cervical spondylosis focus on providing pain relief, lowering the risk of permanent damage, and helping you lead a normal life. Nonsurgical methods are usually very effective.

Physical therapy

Your doctor might send you to a physical therapist for treatment. Physical therapy helps you stretch your neck and shoulder muscles. This makes them stronger and ultimately helps to relieve pain. You might also have neck traction. This involves using weights to increase the space between the cervical joints and relieve the pressure on the cervical discs and nerve roots.

Medications-Over the counter medications
Paracetamol

Paracetamol at full strength (for adults two 500mg tablets four times a day).

Anti-inflammatory painkiller

Some people find these more effective than paracetamol. They can be used in combination with paracetamol. They include ibruprofen or naproxen. Some people with high blood pressure, stomach ulcers, asthma, kidney failure or heart problems may not be able to take anti-inflammatory painkillers.

Codeine

A stronger painkiller such as codeine can be used as an alternative to anti-inflammatories. Codeine is often used to supplement paracetamol.

Low dose trycyclic anti-depressants

A Low dose (10-30mg) trycyclic anti-depressant such as amitriptyline is sometimes used for persistent chronic neck pain.

Your doctor might also prescribe certain medications if over-the-counter drugs don't work. These include:

- muscle relaxants to treat muscle spasms
- narcotics for pain relief
- anti-epileptic drugs to relieve pain caused by nerve damage
- steroid injections, such as prednisolone, to reduce tissue inflammation and subsequently lessen pain
- prescription nonsteroidal anti-inflammatory drugs (NSAIDs), to reduce inflammation

Surgery

If your condition is severe and doesn't respond to other forms of treatment, you might need surgery. This can involve removing bone spurs, parts of your neck bones, or herniated discs to give your spinal cord and nerves more room. Surgery is rarely necessary for cervical spondylosis. However, a doctor may recommend it if the pain is severe and it's affecting your ability to move your arms.

Home treatment options

If your condition is mild, you can try a few things at home to treat it:

- Use a heating pad or a cold pack on your neck to provide pain relief for sore muscles.
- Exercise regularly to help you recover faster.
- Wear a soft neck brace or soft collar to get temporary relief. However, you shouldn't wear a neck brace or collar for long periods of time because that can make your muscles weaker.

****

Organisations providing useful advice and support

www.medwonders.com/support-groups/cervical-spondylosis-degenerative-neck-disease.htm

This online support group for people with cervical spondylosis will help you know more about the disease and get in touch with doctors or other patients.

Healthline

www.healthline.com/health/cervical-spondylosis

NHS Information

www.nhs.uk/conditions/Cervical-spondylosis

Private Treatment

www.nuffieldhealth.com/conditions/cervical-spondylitis

****

Chapter 6

Fibromyalgia

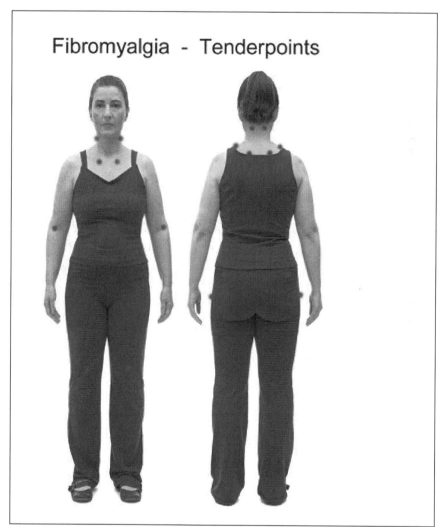

Fibromyalgia - Tenderpoints

Fibromyalgia is a long-term condition that causes considerable pain all over the body. As well as pain, people with fibromyalgia might also experience:

- Heightened sensitivity to pain
- extreme tiredness (fatigue)
- stiffness of the muscles
- difficulty sleeping
- problems known as "fibro-fog", leading to problems with memory and concentration
- frequent headaches
- Irritable Bowel Syndrome (IBS). This is a digestive condition that causes stomach pain and bloating

There is currently no cure for fibromyalgia although there are various treatments to help relieve some of the symptoms and make the condition easier to live with. The treatment available is a combination of medication, for example antidepressants and painkillers, talking therapies, such as cognitive behavioural therapy and counselling and lifestyle changes, such as exercise programmes and relaxation techniques. Exercise in particular has been found to have a number of important benefits for people with fibromyalgia, including helping to reduce pain. See chapter 13 for more on arthritis and exercises.

The causes of fibromyalgia

The exact cause of fibromyalgia is unknown, but it's thought to be related to abnormal levels of certain chemicals in the brain and changes in the way the central nervous system (brain, spinal cord and nerves) processes pain messages carried around the body. It's also thought that there is a genetic link. In some cases, the condition can be triggered by a physically or emotionally stressful event, such as bereavement and giving birth. Anyone can develop fibromyalgia, although it affects more women than men. The condition will usually develop between the ages of 30 and 50, but can occur in people of any age, including young children.

Symptoms of fibromyalgia
The main symptoms of fibromyalgia are:

Pain and sensitivity
You may be sensitive to things like smoke, certain foods and bright lights. Being exposed to something you're sensitive to can cause your other fibromyalgia symptoms to flare up.

Stiffness and tiredness plus poor sleep
Fibromyalgia can make you feel stiff. The stiffness may be most severe when you have been in the same position for a long period of time – for example, when you first wake up in the morning. It can also cause your muscles to spasm, which is when they contract tightly and painfully. Fibromyalgia can also cause extreme tiredness. This can range from a mild tired feeling to the exhaustion often experienced during a flu-like illness. Fibromyalgia can also affect your sleep. You may often wake up tired, even when you have had plenty of sleep. This is because the condition can sometimes prevent you sleeping deeply enough to refresh you properly (this is also described as non-restorative sleep).

Cognitive problems ('fibro-fog')
Cognitive problems are issues related to mental processes, such as thinking and learning. If you have fibromyalgia, you may have:

- trouble remembering and learning new things
- problems with attention and concentration
- slowed or confused speech

Other symptoms

Other symptoms that people with fibromyalgia sometimes experience include:

- dizziness and clumsiness
- feeling too hot or too cold – this is because you're not able to regulate your body temperature properly
- an overwhelming urge to move your legs (restless legs syndrome)
- tingling, numbness, prickling or burning sensations in your hands and feet (pins and needles, also known as paraesthesia)
- in women, unusually painful periods
- anxiety
- depression

Depression

In some cases, having the condition can lead to depression. This is because fibromyalgia can be difficult to deal with, and low levels of certain hormones associated with the condition can make you prone to developing depression.

Causes

It's not clear why some people develop fibromyalgia. The exact cause is unknown, but it's likely that a number of factors are involved, for example abnormal pain messages. The central nervous system (brain, spinal cord and nerves) transmits information all over your body. One of the main theories is that people with fibromyalgia have developed changes in the way the central nervous system processes the pain messages carried around the body. This could be the result of changes to chemicals in the nervous system.

Chemical imbalances

Research has found people with fibromyalgia have abnormally low levels of the hormones serotonin, noradrenaline and dopamine in their brains. Low levels of these hormones may be a key factor in the cause of fibromyalgia, as they're important in regulating things like mood, appetite and sleep. These hormones also play a role in processing pain messges sent by the nerves. Increasing the hormone levels with medication can disrupt these signals.

Sleep problems

It's possible that disturbed sleep patterns may be a cause of fibromyalgia, rather than just a symptom. Fibromyalgia can prevent you sleeping deeply and cause extreme tiredness (fatigue). People with the condition who sleep badly can also have higher levels of pain, suggesting that these sleep problems contribute to the other symptoms of fibromyalgia.

Genetics

Research has suggested genetics may play a small part in the development of fibromyalgia, with some people perhaps more likely than others to develop the condition because of their genes.

Diagnosis

If your GP thinks you may have fibromyalgia, they'll first have to rule out all other conditions that could be causing your symptoms, which is regular procedure. These conditions may include:

- Chronic Fatigue Syndrome-also known as ME– a condition that causes long-term tiredness
- R (chapter 3)
- M – a condition of the central nervous system (the brain and spinal cord) that affects movement and balance

Tests to check for some of these conditions include urine and blood tests, although you may also have X-rays and other scans.

The main criteria for diagnosing fibromyalgia

For fibromyalgia to be diagnosed, certain criteria usually have to be met. The most widely used criteria for a diagnosis are:

- you either have severe pain in 3 to 6 different areas of your body, or you have milder pain in 7 or more different areas
- your symptoms have stayed at a similar level for at least 3 months
- no other reason for your symptoms has been found

Treatment

Your GP will play an important role in your treatment and care. They can help you decide what's best for you, depending on what you prefer and the available treatments. In some cases, several different healthcare professionals may be involved in your care, such as a rheumatologist, a neurologist and a psychologist.

Fibromyalgia has numerous symptoms, meaning that no single treatment will work for all of them. Treatments that work for some people will not necessarily work for others. You may need to try a variety of treatments to find a combination that suits you. This will normally be a combination of medication and also self-help i.e. lifestyle changes.

Medication

You may need to take several different types of medicines for fibromyalgia, including painkillers and antidepressants.

Painkillers

Simple painkillers that are available over the counter from a pharmacy, such as paracetamol, can sometimes help relieve the pain associated with fibromyalgia. However, these are not suitable for everyone, so make sure you read the manufacturer's instructions that come with the medication before using them. If over-the-counter painkillers are not effective, your GP (or another healthcare professional treating you) may prescribe a stronger painkiller, such as codeine or tramadol.

Antidepressants

Antidepressant medication can also help relieve pain for some people with fibromyalgia. They boost the levels of certain chemicals that carry messages to and from the brain, known as neurotransmitters. Low levels of neurotransmitters may be a factor in fibromyalgia, and it's believed that increasing their levels may ease the widespread pain associated with the condition.

There are different types of antidepressants. The choice of medicine largely depends on the severity of your symptoms and any side effects the medicine may cause. Antidepressants used to treat fibromyalgia include:

- tricyclic antidepressants, such as amitriptyline
- serotonin-noradrenaline reuptake inhibitors (SNRIs), such as duloxetine and venlafaxine
- selective serotonin reuptake inhibitors (SSRIs), such as fluoxetine (Prozac) and paroxetine
- A medication called pramipexole, which is not an antidepressant but also affects the levels of neurotransmitters, is sometimes used as well.

Medication to help you sleep

As fibromyalgia can affect your sleeping patterns, you may want medicine to help you sleep. If you're sleeping better, you may find that other symptoms are not as severe. Your GP may recommend an over-the-counter remedy, or prescribe a short course of a stronger medication. Some antidepressants may also improve your sleep quality.

Muscle relaxants

If you have muscle stiffness or spasms (when the muscles contract painfully) as a result of fibromyalgia, your GP may prescribe a short course of a muscle relaxant, such as diazepam. These medicines may also help you sleep better because they can have a sedative effect.

Anticonvulsants

You may also be prescribed an anticonvulsant (anti-seizure) medicine, as these can be effective for those with fibromyalgia. The most commonly used anticonvulsants for fibromyalgia are pregabalin and gabapentin. These are normally used to treat epilepsy, but research has shown they can improve the pain associated with fibromyalgia in some people.

Antipsychotics

Antipsychotic medicines, also called neuroleptics, are sometimes used to help relieve long-term pain

Other treatment options

As well as medication, there are other treatment options that can be used to help cope with the pain of fibromyalgia. These include:

- swimming, sitting or exercising in a heated pool or warm water (known as hydrotherapy or balneotherapy)
- an individually tailored exercise programme
- cognitive behavioural therapy (CBT) – a talking therapy that aims to change the way you think about things, so you can tackle problems more positively
- psychotherapy – a talking therapy that helps you understand and deal with your thoughts and feelings
- relaxation techniques
- psychological support – any kind of counselling or support group that helps you deal with issues caused by fibromyalgia

Alternative therapies

Some people with fibromyalgia try complementary or alternative treatments, such as:

- acupuncture
- massage
- manipulation
- aromatherapy

There's little scientific evidence that such treatments help in the long term. But some people find certain treatments help them relax and feel less stressed, allowing them to cope with their condition better. Research into some complementary medicines, such as plant extracts, has found they're not effective in treating fibromyalgia.

Self help

If you have fibromyalgia, there are several ways to change your lifestyle to help relieve your symptoms and make your condition easier to live with. Your GP, or another healthcare professional treating you, can offer advice and support about making these changes part of your everyday life. There are organisations to support people with fibromyalgia (see end of chapter) that may also be able to offer advice. Below are some tips that may help relieve symptoms of fibromyalgia.

Exercise

Although fatigue is a symptom of fibromyalgia, an exercise programme specially suited to your condition can help you manage your symptoms and improve your overall health. Your GP or physiotherapist may be able to refer you to a health professional who specialises in helping people with fibromyalgia work out an exercise plan. The plan is likely to involve a mixture of aerobic and strengthening exercises.

Pacing yourself

If you have fibromyalgia, it's important to balance periods of activity with periods of rest, not overdoing it or pushing yourself beyond your limits. If you do not pace yourself, it could slow down your progress in the long term. Over time, you can gradually increase your periods of activity while making sure they're balanced with periods of rest.

Relaxation

If you have fibromyalgia, it's important to regularly take time to relax or practise relaxation techniques. Stress can make your symptoms worse or cause them to flare up more often. It could also increase your chances of developing depression. There are many relaxation aids available, including books, tapes and courses, although deep-breathing techniques or meditation may be just as effective. Try to find time each day to do something that relaxes you. Taking time to relax before bed may also help you sleep better at night.

Talking therapies, such as counselling, can also be helpful in combating stress and learning to deal with it effectively. Your GP may recommend you try this as part of your treatment.

Better sleeping habits

Because fibromyalgia can make it difficult to fall asleep or stay asleep it may help to:

- try to get up at the same time every morning

- try to relax before going to bed
- try to create a bedtime routine, such as taking a bath and drinking a warm, milky drink every night
- avoid caffeine, nicotine and alcohol before going to bed
- avoid eating a heavy meal late at night
- make sure your bedroom is a comfortable temperature and is quiet and dark
- avoid checking the time throughout the night

****

Organisations providing useful advice and support

As with other conditions, many people with fibromyalgia find that support groups provide an important network where they can talk to others living with the condition. One of the most well known in this area is:

Fibromyalgia Action UK

Helpline on 0300 999 3333

www.fmauk.org

Fibromyalgia Action UK is a charity that offers information and support to people with fibromyalgia. The charity also has a network of local support groups you may find helpful and a online community, where you can find out about news, events and ongoing research into the condition.

Another support group you may find useful is

UK Fibromyalgia

7 Ashbourne Road
Bournemouth, Dorset, BH5 2JS

Email Address:info@ukfibromyalgia.com

ukfibromyalgia.com

****

Chapter 7

Lupus

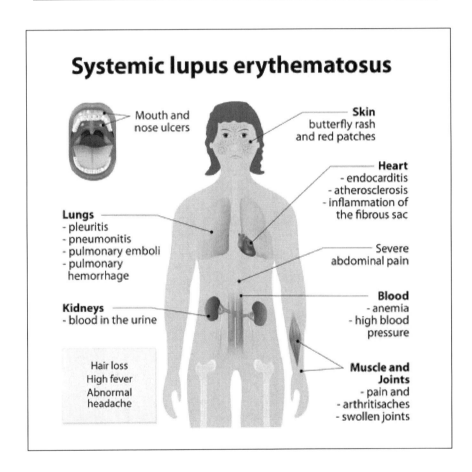

Systemic lupus erythematosus

Mouth and nose ulcers

Skin
butterfly rash
and red patches

Heart
- endocarditis
- atherosclerosis
- inflammation of
  the fibrous sac

Lungs
- pleuritis
- pneumonitis
- pulmonary emboli
- pulmonary
  hemorrhage

Severe
abdominal pain

Kidneys
- blood in the urine

Blood
- anemia
- high blood
  pressure

Hair loss
High fever
Abnormal
headache

Muscle and
Joints
- pain and
- arthritisaches
- swollen joints

What is lupus?

Lupus, a form of arthritis, is a chronic autoimmune disease that causes inflammation throughout your body. An autoimmune disease is a condition in which your body's own immune system is responsible for the inflammation and breakdown of its own cells. The inflammation seen in lupus can affect various organs and tissues in your body, including your:

- joints
- skin
- heart
- blood
- lung
- brain
- kidneys

This disease can be severe and potentially life-threatening. It can cause permanent organ damage. However, many people with lupus experience a mild version of it. Currently, there's no known cure for lupus.

What are the lupus types?

Doctors usually categorize four lupus types. These include:

Systemic lupus erythematosus (see main diagram): The most common lupus type, this condition can range from mild to severe. The condition causes symptoms that may get worse over time, then improve.

Cutaneous lupus: This type of lupus is generally limited to your skin. It may cause rashes and permanent lesions with scarring. The cutaneous form of skin lupus that causes scarring is called discoid lupus.

DILE: Long-term use of certain prescription medications can lead to drug-induced lupus. DILE is caused by the long-term use of certain prescribed medications. It mimics the symptoms of systemic lupus, but in most cases, the condition doesn't affect major organs.

Neonatal lupus: This condition is extremely rare and affects infants whose mothers have lupus. Symptoms of this condition may include a skin rash, low blood cell counts, and liver problems after birth. While some babies may have heart defects, most have symptoms that will go away after several months.

Some lupus types have further divisions depending on a person's symptoms.

What are the symptoms of lupus?

The symptoms of lupus vary according to the parts of your body affected. Symptoms can disappear suddenly. They can be permanent or flare up occasionally. Although no two cases of lupus are the same, the most common symptoms and signs include:

- a fever
- fatigue
- body aches
- joint pain
- rashes, including a butterfly rash on the face
- skin lesions
- shortness of breath
- chronic dry eyes
- chest pain
- headaches
- confusion
- memory loss

Some of the later symptoms of lupus include kidney problems due to inflammation. A person may experience high blood pressure, dark urine, and blood in the urine.

What are the causes of lupus?

While doctors don't know exactly what causes lupus, they think it may be a combination of many underlying factors. These include:

Environment: Doctors have identified potential triggers like smoking, stress, and exposure to toxins like silica dust as potential lupus causes.

Genetics: Having a family history of lupus may put a person at slightly higher risk for experiencing the condition.

Hormones: Some studies suggest that abnormal hormone levels, such as increased estrogen levels, could contribute to lupus.

Infections: Doctors are still studying the link between infections like cytomegalovirus, Epstein-Barr, or hepatitis C and causes of lupus.

Medications: Long-term use of certain medications.

It's also possible a person has experienced none of the known potential causes of lupus listed here and yet has the condition.

What are the risk factors for lupus?

Examples of risk factors for lupus include:

- being a woman
- being between the ages of 15 and 44
- being a member of certain ethnic groups

Having a family history of lupus

Having risk factors for lupus in terms of family history doesn't mean you will get lupus, but that you are at increased risk compared to those who don't have family risk factors.

Is lupus curable?

Currently, there is no cure for lupus. An estimated 80 to 90 percent of people living with lupus can live a normal life span with treatment and follow-up. However, research regularly explores promising innovations in lupus treatment. These include some animal studies that show early promise that lupus is curable.

While there is no cure for lupus at this time, you can take medications to control lupus symptoms. Examples of lupus treatment medications include:

- nonsteroidal anti-inflammatory drugs (NSAIDs)
- antimalarial medications
- DHEA, a male hormone that may reduce some lupus effects, such as hair loss
- corticosteroids
- immunosuppressive drugs

A doctor will consider a person's lupus symptoms and their severity when recommending lupus treatments. Doctors may also recommend lifestyle changes, such as avoiding excess ultraviolet sunlight exposure. Some people take supplements in addition to their medications to reduce lupus symptoms. Examples of these supplements include flax seed, fish oil, and vitamin D.

Is there a lupus diet?

Doctors haven't established a definitive lupus diet. However, there are some foods that those with lupus should usually avoid, mostly due to the medications they typically take. Examples include alcohol, which interacts negatively with many NSAIDs and can cause gastrointestinal bleeding.

Avoiding foods high in salt and cholesterol not only is beneficial for a person's health, but also helps to prevent bloating due to corticosteroid use. Other healthy steps to reduce inflammation in the body for those with lupus include:

- fish high in omega-3 fatty acids, such as salmon, tuna, or mackerel
- foods high in calcium, such as low-fat dairy products
- eating whole-grain carbohydrate sources
- eating a blend of colourful fruits and vegetables

However, people with lupus should avoid alfalfa. This is because the amino acid known as L-canavanine found in alfalfa sprouts and seeds may increase inflammation and lead to lupus flare-ups. See chapter 13 for more advice about diet and arthritis generally.

How do doctors make a lupus diagnosis?

Doctors don't have a specific blood test or imaging study to use to diagnose lupus. Instead, they consider a person's signs and symptoms and rule out other potential conditions that could be causing a person's symptoms. In addition to taking a detailed medical history and physical examination, doctors may perform the following tests to diagnose lupus:

Laboratory tests: These could include a complete blood count (CBC), a test doctors use to determine the number and type of red blood cells, white blood cells, and platelets in the blood. Other tests a doctor may order include an erythrocyte sedimentation rate, protein levels, and anti-nuclear antibody test, which can indicate heightened immune system activity.

Imaging tests: Chest X-rays and echocardiograms are two imaging studies that may indicate the buildup of fluid on or around the heart. Positive results may reflect lupus causes.

Tissue biopsy: Doctors can take a biopsy or sample of cells from an area of lupus-like rash to determine if cells typical of a person with lupus are present. A doctor may also perform a kidney biopsy to see if the kidneys appear damaged due to lupus.

Life expectancy with lupus

Medical innovations and improvements in diagnostic testing have meant people with lupus are living longer than ever. An estimated 80% to 90% of people diagnosed with lupus will live a normal life span. Those who have severe lupus symptoms or who experience a severe flare-up are at greater risk for complications than those with mild to moderate lupus.

Are there lupus prevention tips?

For most lupus types, the condition isn't preventable. An exception is the medications known to cause drug-induced lupus. However, it's important a person discuss the risks and benefits as not taking these medications could also result in life-threatening effects. Additionally, a person may wish to engage in preventive measures that reduce the likelihood they will experience a lupus flare-up. These include:

Avoiding direct sunlight: Excess sun exposure can cause a lupus-related rash. A person should always wear sunscreen when going outdoors and avoid direct sunlight when the sun's rays are most overhead, which is usually between 10 a.m. and 4 p.m.

Practicing stress management techniques. These include meditation, yoga, or massages that can help a person relieve stress whenever possible.

Practicing infection prevention techniques. This includes frequent hand-washing and avoiding being around those with colds and other illnesses.

Getting plenty of rest. Rest is vital in helping a person's body to heal.

****

Organisations providing useful advice and support

Lupus UK
St James House
Eastern Road
Romford
Essex RM1 3NH
England
Tel: 01708 731251
www.lupusuk.org.uk

LUPUS UK is the only national registered charity supporting people with systemic lupus and discoid lupus and assisting those approaching diagnosis. They presently have over 5500 Members and a number of Regional Groups around the UK who arrange medical talks, publish local newsletters, set up local occasions and organise fundraising events.

LUPUS UK also produces an informative national magazine with lupus articles, letters, reports, and photographs, and operates a strong Grant Programme for research purposes and welfare.

Online support
mylupusteam.com

Extract from their website:

"MyLupusTeam is a free social network that makes it easy for you to:

- get the emotional support you need from others like you, and
- gain practical advice and insights on managing treatment or therapies for lupus

When you or a loved one are first diagnosed, it's not uncommon to feel alone and uncertain of where to find the best information and people that can help you now. We believe in making it easy to find the best people around you to help you get the answers you need, and to find support from people who can truly relate. The main currency on our site is trust – the more you share in posts and your stories, the more questions you ask and answer, the more your support will be valued by other members.

MyLupusTeam is the only social network where you can truly connect, make real friendships, and share daily ups and downs in a judgment-free place".

There are numerous other online support groups, many in the USA, which offer very useful advice and support.

****

Chapter 8

Gout

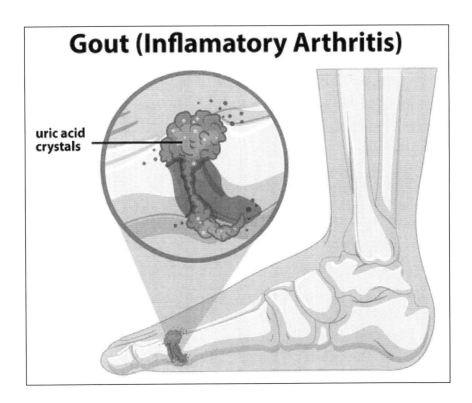

Gout (Inflamatory Arthritis)

uric acid crystals

About gout

Many people, at some time in their lives, suffer from Gout, in one form or another, It is very painful.

Gout is a type of arthritis in which small crystals form inside and around the joints. It causes sudden attacks of severe pain and swelling. Gout, otherwise known as uric acid arthropathy, is a rheumatic complaint, which usually attacks a single joint at a time. There are two types of gout, as below.

Primary hyperurcaemia and gout. Hyperuricaemia means an increased level of uric acid in the blood. Its usually caused by an hereditary abnormality in the system, which changes the nucleic acid into uric acid. In this case, the body is incapable of excreting uric acid fast enough.

Secondary hyperuricaemia and gout.
This is caused by another disease or because of complications. In these cases, the problem is that the body produces such large quantities of uric acid that consumption of certain medicines (e.g. diuretic preparations, which increase the output of urine) mean that the kidneys cannot keep up.

It's estimated that between one and two in every 100 people in the UK are affected by gout which can be extremely painful and debilitating, but treatments are available to help. The condition mainly affects men over 30 and women after the menopause.

Signs and symptoms of gout
Any joint can be affected by gout, but more commonly it affects joints towards the ends of the limbs, such as the toes, ankles, knees and fingers. Signs and symptoms of gout include:

- severe pain in one or more joints
- the joint feeling hot and very tender
- swelling in and around the affected joint
- red, shiny skin over the affected joint

Symptoms develop rapidly over a few hours and typically last three to 10 days. After this time the pain should pass and the joint should return to normal. The first gout attack is often at night. Typically the affected person will wake up in the middle of the night with extreme pain near the joint of the big toe or pain in the knee. Even the smallest stimuli, such as a blanket on the toe can cause pain.

Almost everyone with gout will experience further attacks at some point, usually within a year.

When to see your GP
See your GP if you suspect you have gout and it hasn't been previously diagnosed, particularly if the pain keeps getting worse and you also have a high temperature (fever). It's important that a diagnosis is confirmed because other conditions that require urgent treatment, such as an infected joint, can sometimes cause similar symptoms.

How does the doctor diagnose gout?
- The diagnosis is usually made from the way the patient presents the symptoms, plus the clinical picture.
- In order to rule out other rheumatic complaints, the doctor will usually take a blood sample to measure the concentration of uric acid. He may also undertake an X-ray examination and an examination of the synovial fluid (found within joints), where uric crystals will be visible.

What causes gout?

As we have seen gout is caused by a build-up of a substance called uric acid in the blood. If you produce too much uric acid or your kidneys don't filter enough out, it can build up and cause tiny sharp crystals to form in and around joints. These crystals can cause the joint to become inflamed (red and swollen) and painful. Things that may increase your chances of getting gout include:

- obesity, high blood pressure and/or diabetes
- having a close relative with gout
- kidney problems
- eating foods that cause a build-up of uric acid, such as red meat, offal and seafood
- drinking too much beer or spirits

Treatments for gout

If you have gout, treatment is available from your GP to:

- relieve symptoms during an attack— this can be done using ice packs and by taking medications such as non-steroidal anti-inflammatory drugs (NSAIDs), colchicine or corticosteroids
- prevent further attacks through a combination of lifestyle changes, such as losing weight or changing your diet, and taking medication that lowers uric acid levels, such as allopurinol

With treatment, many people are able to reduce their uric acid levels sufficiently to dissolve the crystals that cause gout – and as a result have no further attacks. However, lifelong treatment is usually required.

Sometimes gout can lead to further problems, particularly if it's left untreated. These can include:

- kidney stones
- small firm lumps of uric acid crystals under the skin called tophi
- permanent joint damage

Kidney stones

Uric acid crystals can cause a build up of stones in your kidneys. Often, the stones are small and are passed in your urine. Sometimes, they can become too large to pass and block parts of your urinary tract. Symptoms of kidney stones include:

- pain or aching in your lower back, side, abdomen, or groin
- nausea
- increased urge to urinate
- pain when urinating
- difficulty urinating
- blood in your urine
- foul-smelling urine

If you also have a kidney infection, you may experience fever or chills.

Tophaceous gout

If you've had hyperuricemia for several years, uric acid crystals can form clumps called tophi. These hard lumps are found under your skin, around your joints, and in the curve at the top of your ear. Tophi can worsen joint pain and over time damage your joints or compress your nerves. They're often visible to the eye and can become disfiguring.

What to avoid:

- red meats
- sugary foods and beverages, especially if they contain high-fructose corn syrup
- organ meat, such as liver
- meat gravies
- some seafood, such as anchovies, sardines, scallops, and mussels
- fish, such as tuna, cod, herring, and haddock
- spinach, peas, and mushrooms
- beans and lentils
- oatmeal
- wheat germ and bran
- beer and alcoholic beverages
- yeast supplements

If you can't avoid the above altogether then you should take in small doses.

****

Organisations providing useful advice and support

The UK Gout Society

UK Gout Society Secretariat

PO Box 90

Hindhead

GU27 9FW

www.ukgoutsociety.org

The UK Gout Society is a registered charity and was established in 2002 to provide basic information to people living with gout, their families, friends and carers - and increase public awareness about this painful, potentially disabling, but very treatable, disorder. Their trustee board comprises experienced rheumatologists and health professionals working in the field of gout.

The UK Gout Society is a member of ARMA (Arthritis and Musculoskeletal Alliance) - the umbrella body providing a collective voice for the arthritis and musculoskeletal community in the UK. http://arma.uk.net/

Online groups
Health Forum
https://ehealthforum.com/health/gout.html
Extract from their website:
"Welcome to the Gout Forum - a health community featuring member and doctor discussions ranging from a specific symptom to related conditions, treatment options, medication, side effects, diet, and emotional issues surrounding medical conditions.

Chapter 9

Psoriatic Arthritis

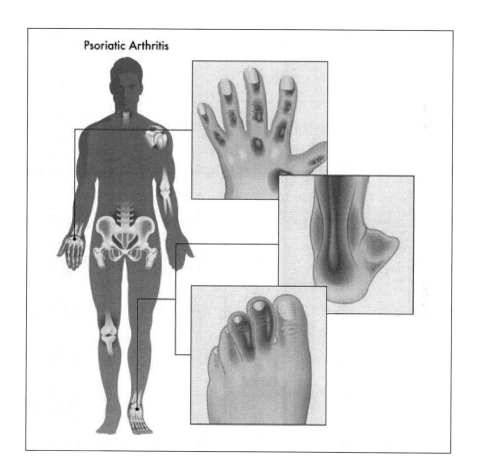

Psoriatic Arthritis

Psoriatic arthritis

Psoriatic arthritis is a type of arthritis that develops in some people with the skin condition psoriasis. It typically causes affected joints to become inflamed, stiff and painful.

Like psoriasis, psoriatic arthritis is a long-term condition that can get progressively worse. In severe cases, there's a risk of the joints becoming permanently damaged or deformed, which may require surgical treatment.

However, with an early diagnosis and appropriate treatment, it's possible to slow down the progression of the condition and minimise or prevent permanent damage to the joints.

Symptoms of psoriatic arthritis

The pain, swelling and stiffness associated with psoriatic arthritis can affect any joint in the body, but the condition often affects the hands, feet, knees, neck, spine and elbows. The severity of the condition can vary considerably from person to person. Some people may have severe problems affecting many joints, whereas others may only notice mild symptoms in 1 or 2 joints.

There may be times when your symptoms improve and periods when they get worse (known as flare-ups or relapses). Relapses can be very difficult to predict, but can often be managed with medication when they do occur.

When to seek medical advice

See your GP if you experience persistent pain, swelling or stiffness in your joints – even if you haven't been diagnosed with psoriasis.

If you've been diagnosed with psoriasis, you should have check-ups at least once a year to monitor your condition. Make sure you let your doctor know if you're experiencing any problems with your joints.

Causes of psoriatic arthritis

Between 1 and 2 in every 5 people with psoriasis develop psoriatic arthritis. It usually develops within 10 years of psoriasis being diagnosed, although some people may experience problems with their joints before they notice any symptoms affecting their skin. Like psoriasis, psoriatic arthritis is thought to occur as a result of the immune system mistakenly attacking healthy tissue. However, it's not clear why some people with psoriasis develop psoriatic arthritis and others don't.

Diagnosing psoriatic arthritis

If your doctor thinks you may have arthritis, they should refer you to a rheumatologist for an assessment. The British Association of Dermatologists website has information on the psoriasis epidemiology screening tool (PEST) (PDF, 209kb). This is a questionnaire you may be asked to fill out, which helps your doctor decide if you need a referral. People with psoriasis should be asked to fill this out annually.

A rheumatologist will usually be able to diagnose psoriatic arthritis if you have psoriasis and problems with your joints. They'll also try to rule out other types of arthritis, such as rheumatoid arthritis and osteoarthritis.

A number of tests may be carried out to help confirm a diagnosis, including:

- Blood tests to check for signs of inflammation in your body and the presence of certain antibodies found in other types of arthritis
- X-rays or scans of your joints

Treating psoriatic arthritis

The main aims of treatment will be to relieve your symptoms, slow the progression of the condition and improve your quality of life. For most people, this involves trying a number of different medications, some of which can also treat the psoriasis. Ideally, you should take one medication to treat both your psoriasis and psoriatic arthritis whenever possible. The main medications used to treat psoriatic arthritis are summarised below and include:

- non-steroidal anti-inflammatory drugs (NSAIDs)
- corticosteroids
- disease-modifying anti-rheumatic drugs (DMARDs)
- biological therapies

Non-steroidal anti-inflammatory drugs (NSAIDs)

Your GP may first prescribe non-steroidal anti-inflammatory drugs (NSAIDs) to see if they help relieve pain and reduce inflammation. There are two types of NSAIDs and they work in slightly different ways:

- traditional NSAIDs, such as ibuprofen, naproxen or diclofenac
- COX-2 inhibitors (often called coxibs), such as celecoxib or etoricoxib

Like all medications, NSAIDs can have side effects. Your doctor will take precautions to reduce the risk of these, such as prescribing the lowest dose necessary to control your symptoms for the shortest time possible. If side effects do occur, they usually affect the stomach and intestines, and can include indigestion and stomach ulcers. A medication called a proton pump inhibitor (PPI) will often be prescribed alongside NSAIDs – a PPI helps protect your stomach by reducing the amount of acid it produces.

If NSAIDs alone aren't helpful, some of the medications below may be recommended.

Corticosteroids

Like NSAIDs, corticosteroids can help reduce pain and swelling. If you have a single inflamed or swollen joint, your doctor may inject the medication directly into the joint. This can offer rapid relief with minimal side effects, and the effect can last from a few weeks to several months. Corticosteroids can also be taken as a tablet, or as an injection into the muscle, to help lots of joints. However, doctors are generally cautious about this because the medication can cause significant side effects if used in the long term, and psoriasis can flare up when you stop using it.

Disease-modifying anti-rheumatic drugs (DMARDs)

Disease-modifying anti-rheumatic drugs (DMARDs) are medications that work by tackling the underlying causes of the inflammation in your joints. They can help to ease your symptoms and slow the progression of psoriatic arthritis. The earlier you start taking a DMARD, the more effective it will be.

Leflunomide is often the first drug given for psoriatic arthritis, although sulfasalazine or methotrexate may be considered as alternatives. It can take several weeks or months to notice a DMARD working, so it's important to keep taking the medication, even if it doesn't seem to be working at first.

Biological treatments

Biological treatments are a newer form of treatment for psoriatic arthritis. You may be offered one of these treatments if:

- your psoriatic arthritis hasn't responded to at least two different types of DMARD
- you're not able to be treated with at least two different types of DMARD

Biological drugs work by stopping particular chemicals in the blood from activating your immune system to attack the lining of your joints.

Some of the biological medicines you may be offered include:

- adalimumab
- apremilast
- certolizumab
- etanercept
- golimumab
- infliximab
- secukinumab
- ustekinumab
- ixekizumab
- tofacitinib

The most common side effect of biological treatments is a reaction in the area of skin where the medication is injected, such as redness, swelling or pain, although these reactions aren't usually serious. However, biological treatments can sometimes cause other side effects, including problems with your liver, kidneys or blood count, so you'll usually need to have regular blood or urine tests to check for these.

Biological treatments can also make you more likely to develop infections.

Tell your doctor as soon as possible if you develop symptoms of an infection, such as:

- a sore throat
- a high temperature (fever)
- diarrhoea

Biological medication will usually be recommended for three months at first, to see if it helps. If it's effective, the medication can be continued. Otherwise, your doctor may suggest stopping the medication or swapping to an alternative biological treatment.

Complementary therapies

There's not enough scientific evidence to say that complementary therapies, such as balneotherapy (bathing in water containing minerals), works in treating psoriatic arthritis. also not enough evidence to support taking any kind of food supplement as treatment. Complementary therapies can sometimes react with other treatments, so talk to your GP, specialist or pharmacist if you're thinking of using any.

Managing related conditions

As with psoriasis and other types of inflammatory arthritis, you may be more likely to get some other conditions – such as cardiovascular disease (CVD) – if you have psoriatic arthritis. CVD is the term for conditions of the heart or blood vessels, such as heart disease and stroke.Your doctor should carry out tests each year (such as blood pressure and cholesterol tests) so they can check whether you have CVD and offer additional treatment, if necessary.You can also help yourself by:

- having a good balance between rest and regular physical activity

- losing weight, if you are overweight

- not smoking

- only drinking moderate amounts of alcohol

Your care team

As well as your GP and a rheumatologist, you may also be cared for by:

- a specialist nurse – who will often be your first point of contact with your specialist care team

- a dermatologist (skin specialist) – who will be responsible for treating your psoriasis symptoms

- a physiotherapist – who can devise an exercise plan to keep your joints mobile

- an occupational therapist – who can identify any problems you have in everyday activities and find ways to overcome or manage these

- a psychologist – who can offer psychological support if you need it

****

Organisations providing useful advice and support

Psoriasis Association

www.psoriasis-association.org.uk/psoriasis-and-treatments

The Psoriasis Association is the leading national charity and membership organisation for people affected by psoriasis in the UK. Through their work, they help people whose lives are affected by psoriasis and psoriatic arthritis. They do this through funding research, providing information and raising awareness.

What they Do

- They offer good quality, reliable and independent information and advice.
- They raise awareness of psoriasis and work with key health officials on strategic issues.
- They distribute copies of their members' magazine 'Pso' to all Dermatology and Rheumatology departments in the UK.
- They represent the interests of members at a local and national level
- They fund and promote research into the causes, nature and care of people with psoriasis.

NHS

www.nhs.uk/conditions/Psoriasis

****

Chapter 10

Reactive Arthritis

Reactive arthritis is a condition that causes redness and swelling (inflammation) in various joints in the body, especially the knees, feet, toes, hips and ankles. It usually develops after you've had an infection, particularly a sexually transmitted infection or food poisoning. In most cases, it clears up within a few months and causes no long-term problems. Men and women of any age can get it, but it's more common in men, and people aged between 20 and 40.

Symptoms of reactive arthritis

The most common symptom of reactive arthritis is pain, stiffness and swelling in the joints and tendons, most commonly the knees, feet, toes, hips and ankles. In some people it can also affect the:

- genital tract – causing pain when peeing, or discharge from the penis or vagina
- eyes – causing eye pain, redness, sticky discharge, conjunctivitis and, rarely, inflammation of the eye (iritis)

Most people will not get all the above symptoms. They can come on suddenly but usually start to develop a few days after you get an infection somewhere else in your body.

Causes of reactive arthritis

Typically, reactive arthritis is caused by a sexually transmitted infection (STI), such as chlamydia, or an infection of the bowel, such as food poisoning. You may also develop reactive arthritis if you, or someone close to you, has recently had glandular fever or slapped cheek syndrome. The body's immune system seems to overreact to the infection and starts attacking healthy tissue, causing it to become inflamed. But the exact reason for this is unknown. People who have a gene called HLA-B27 are much more likely to develop reactive arthritis than those who don't, but it's unclear why.

When to see your GP

If you have symptoms of reactive arthritis, you should see your GP, especially if you have recently had symptoms of an infection – such as diarrhoea, or pain when peeing. There's no single test for reactive arthritis, although blood and urine tests, genital swabs, ultrasound scans and X-rays may be used to check for infection and rule out other causes of your symptoms. Your GP will also want to know about your recent medical history, such as whether you may have recently had a bowel infection or an STI.

If you think you might have an STI, you can also visit a local genitourinary medicine (GUM) clinic or other sexual health service. These clinics can often see you straight away, without a GP referral.

If your GP thinks you have reactive arthritis, they may refer you to a rheumatologist. They may also refer you to a specialist if you have problems with your eyes.

Treatment for reactive arthritis

Treatment usually focuses on:

- using antibiotics to clear any STI that may have triggered the reactive arthritis
- using painkillers such as ibuprofen to relieve joint pain and stiffness
- managing any severe or ongoing arthritis, usually using medications such as steroids or disease-modifying anti-rheumatic drugs (DMARDs)
- Most people start returning to normal activities after 3 to 6 months. Symptoms don't usually last longer than 12 months. The main, and sometimes only, symptom of reactive arthritis is pain, stiffness and swelling in the joints and tendons

Joint symptoms

Reactive arthritis can affect any joints, but it's most common in the knees, feet, toes, hips and ankles. Symptoms include:

- pain, tenderness and swelling in your joints
- pain and tenderness in some tendons, especially at the heels
- pain in your lower back and buttocks
- sausage-like swelling of your fingers and toes
- joint stiffness – particularly in the morning

Genital tract symptoms

Sometimes, you can also have symptoms of a urinary tract infection. These include:

- needing to pee suddenly, or more often than usual

- pain or a burning sensation when peeing
- smelly or cloudy pee
- blood in your pee
- pain in your lower tummy
- feeling tired and unwell

Eye symptoms

Occasionally, you may get inflammation of the eyes (conjunctivitis or, rarely, iritis). Symptoms can include:

- red eyes
- watery eyes
- eye pain
- swollen eyelids
- sensitivity to light

This could be a symptom of iritis – and the sooner you get treatment, the more successful it is likely to be.

Other symptoms

Reactive arthritis can also cause:

- flu-like symptoms
- a high temperature (fever)
- weight loss
- mouth ulcers
- a scaly rash on the hands or feet

Most people will make a full recovery within a year, but a small number of people experience long-term joint problems. Treatment usually focuses on:

- clearing the original infection that triggered the reactive arthritis – usually using antibiotics in the case of sexually transmitted infections (STIs)
- relieving symptoms such as pain and stiffness – usually using painkillers such as ibuprofen
- managing severe or ongoing reactive arthritis – usually using medications such as steroids or disease-modifying anti-rheumatic drugs (DMARDs)

Antibiotics
Antibiotics will not treat reactive arthritis itself but are sometimes prescribed if you have an ongoing infection – particularly if you have an STI. Your recent sexual partner(s) may also need treatment.

Non-steroidal anti-inflammatory drugs
Anti-inflammatory painkillers (NSAIDs), such as ibuprofen, can be taken to reduce inflammation and relieve pain.

Steroid medication
If you have severe inflammation, or you can't take NSAIDs or they didn't work for you, you may be prescribed steroid medication to reduce inflammation. Steroids may be given as tablets if several of your joints are affected. If only one or two joints are affected, steroids may be injected directly into the affected joint or tendon.

Disease-modifying anti-rheumatic drugs (DMARDs)
If your symptoms don't get better after a few weeks with other treatment or are very severe, you may be prescribed a DMARD,

which also work by reducing inflammation. They may be prescribed on their own but can also be prescribed in combination with steroids or NSAIDs, or with both. The most commonly used DMARDs are methotrexate and sulfasalazine.

It can take a few months before you notice a DMARD is working, so it's important to keep taking it even if you don't see immediate results. Common side effects of methotrexate and sulfasalazine include feeling sick, diarrhoea, loss of appetite and headaches, although these usually improve once your body gets used to the medication. DMARDs may also cause changes in your blood or liver, so it's important to have regular blood tests while taking these medicines.

Other drugs

If your reactive arthritis is very severe, even stronger drugs, known as biologics, may be prescribed. These have to be given regularly by injection and may increase your risk of getting infections.

Self-care

There are also things you can do yourself to relieve your symptoms. When you first start getting symptoms of reactive arthritis, you should try to get plenty of rest and avoid using the affected joints. As your symptoms improve, you should begin to do exercises to stretch and strengthen the affected muscles, and improve the range of movement in your affected joints. Your GP or specialist may recommend exercises for your arthritis. Alternatively, you may be referred for physiotherapy.

You might also find ice packs and heat pads useful in reducing joint pain and swelling. Wrap them in a clean towel before putting them against your skin. Splints, heel pads and shoe inserts (insoles) may also help.

How to stop reactive arthritis coming back

There is a risk you could develop reactive arthritis again if you get another infection. The best way to avoid this is by protecting yourself against STIs and bowel infections.

The most effective way of preventing STIs is to always use a barrier method of contraception, such as a condom, during sex with a new partner. Ensuring good standards of hygiene when preparing and storing food can help to prevent bowel infections.

****

Organisations providing useful advice and support

Arthritis Care
www.arthritiscare.org.uk/Reactivearthritisfactsheet2015

Arthritis care publishes a very useful factsheet concerning Reactive Arthritis. For confidential information and support, contact the Arthritis Care Helpline Freephone: 0808 800 4050 10am-4pm (weekdays) Email: Helplines@arthritiscare.org.uk

For information about Arthritis Care and the services they offer, contact them at: www.arthritiscare.org.uk Arthritis Care UK office and England regional services: Tel: 020 7380 6500

Arthritis Care in Northern Ireland Tel: 028 9078 2940 Email: NIreland@arthritiscare.org.uk

Arthritis Care in Scotland Tel: 0141 954 7776 Email: Scotland@arthritiscare.org.uk

Arthritis Care in Wales Tel: 029 2044 4155 Email: Wales@arthritiscare.org.uk

NHS
www.nhs.uk/conditions/reactive-arthritis/treatment

****

Chapter 11

Polymyalgia Rheumatica

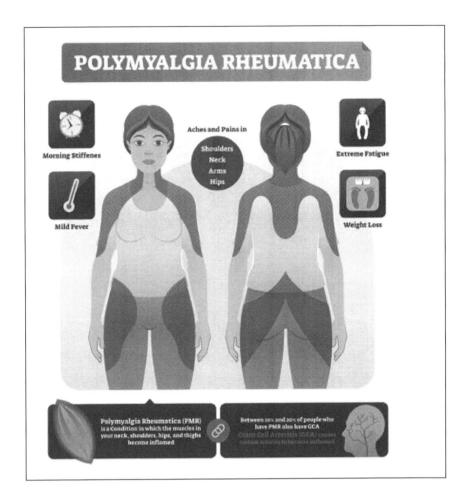

Polymyalgia rheumatica (PMR) is a syndrome with pain or stiffness, usually in the neck, shoulders, upper arms, and hips, but which may occur all over the body. The pain can be very sudden, or can occur gradually over a period. Most people with PMR wake up in the morning with pain in their muscles. However, cases have occurred in which the person has developed the pain during the evenings or has pain and stiffness all day long.

People who have polymyalgia rheumatica may also have temporal arteritis , an inflammation of blood vessels in the face which can cause blindness if not treated quickly. The pain and stiffness can lead to a reduced quality of life, and can also lead to depression. It is thought to be brought on by a viral or bacterial illness or trauma of some kind, but genetics does play a factor as well.

PMR is usually treated with corticosteroids taken by mouth. Most people need to continue the corticosteroid treatment for two to three years. PMR sometimes goes away on its own in a year or two, but medications and self-care measures can improve the rate of recovery.

Signs and Symptoms of Polymialgia Rheumatica

A wide range of symptoms can indicate if a person has polymyalgia rheumatica. The classic symptoms include:

- Pain and stiffness (moderate to severe) in the neck, shoulders, upper arms, thighs, and hips, which inhibits activity, especially in the morning/after sleeping. Pain can also occur in the groin area and in the buttocks. The pain can be limited to one of these areas as well. It is a disease of the "girdles" meaning shoulder girdle or pelvic girdle.
- Fatigue and lack of appetite (possibly leading to weight loss) are also indicative of polymyalgia rheumatica.
- Anaemia

- An overall feeling of illness or flu-like symptoms.
- Low-grade (mild) fever or abnormal temperature is sometimes present.

Causes

The cause of PMR is not well understood. The pain and stiffness result from the activity of inflammatory cells and proteins that are normally a part of the body's disease-fighting immune system, and the inflammatory activity seems to be concentrated in tissues surrounding the affected joints. During this disorder, the white blood cells in the body attack the lining of the joints, causing inflammation. Inherited factors also play a role in the probability that an individual will develop PMR. Several theories have included viral stimulation of the immune system in genetically susceptible individuals.

Infectious disease may be a contributing factor. This would be expected with sudden onset of symptoms, for example. In addition, new cases often appear in cycles in the general population, implying a viral connection. The viruses thought to be involved include the adenovirus, which causes respiratory infections; the human parvovirus B19, an infection that affects children; and the human parainfluenza virus. In addition, sufferers attribute the onset of PMR to stress.

Diagnosis

No specific test exists to diagnose polymyalgia rheumatica; many other diseases can cause inflammation and pain in muscles, but a few tests can help narrow down the cause of the pain. Limitation in shoulder motion, or swelling of the joints in the wrists or hands, are noted by the doctor. A patient's answers to questions, a general physical exam, and the results of tests can help a doctor determine the cause of pain and stiffness.

One blood test usually performed is the erythrocyte sedimentation rate (ESR) which measures how fast the patient's red blood cells settle in a test tube. The faster the blood cells settle, the higher the ESR value, which means inflammation is present. Many conditions can cause an elevated ESR, so this test alone is not proof that a person has polymyalgia rheumatica.

Another test that checks the level of C-reactive protein (CRP) in the blood may also be conducted. CRP is produced by the liver in response to an injury or infection, and people with polymyalgia rheumatica usually have high levels. However, like the ESR, this test is also not very specific.

Treatment

Prednisolone (Steroid) is the drug of choice for PMR, and treatment duration is frequently greater than one year. If the patient does not experience dramatic improvement after three days of 10–20 mg oral prednisolone per day, the diagnosis is usually reconsidered. Sometimes relief of symptoms occurs in only several hours.

Side effects of prednisolone

About 1 in 20 people who take prednisolone will experience changes in their mental state when they take the medication. You may feel depressed and suicidal, anxious or confused. Some people also experience hallucinations, which is seeing or hearing things that aren't there. Contact your GP as soon as possible if you experience changes to your mental state. Other side effects of prednisolone include:

- increased appetite, which often leads to weight gain
- increased blood pressure
- mood changes, such as becoming aggressive or irritable with people
- weakening of the bones (osteoporosis)
- stomach ulcers
- increased risk of infection, particularly with the varicella-zoster virus, the virus that causes chickenpox and shingles

You should seek immediate medical advice if you think you've been exposed to the varicella-zoster virus or if a member of your household develops chickenpox or shingles. The risk of these side effects should improve as your dose of prednisolone is decreased.

Nonsteroidal anti-inflammatory drugs (NSAIDs) such as ibuprofen are ineffective in the initial treatment of PMR, but they may be used in conjunction with the maintenance dose of corticosteroid. Along with medical treatment, patients are encouraged to exercise and eat healthily—helping to maintain a strong immune system and build strong muscles and bones. A diet of fruits, vegetables, whole grains, and low-fat meat and dairy products, avoiding foods with high levels of refined sugars and salt is recommended. See chapter 13 on diet.

The circumstances are not certain as to why an individual will get polymyalgia rheumatica, but a few factors show a relationship with the disorder:

- Usually, PMR only affects adults over the age of 50.
- The average age of a person who has PMR is about 70 years old.

- Women are twice as likely to get PMR as men.
- Caucasians are more likely to get this disease. It is more likely to affect people of Northern European origin; Scandinavians are especially vulnerable.
- About 50% of people with temporal arteritis also have polymyalgia rheumatica.

****

Organisations providing useful advice and support

Polymyalgia Rheumatica and Giant Cell Arteritis (PMRGCAUK)

PMRGCAuk is a registered charity set up to meet the needs of people with these debilitating conditions, their friends, family and helping professionals.

Helpline 0300 111 5090 or email helpline@pmrgca.org.uk

Online community

The site also has an online support group.

General advice and support sites

NHS

www.nhs.uk/conditions/Polymyalgia-rheumatica

Healthline

www.healthline.com/health/polymyalgia-rheumatica

Versus Arthritis (formerly Arthritis UK and Arthritis Research UK)

www.versusarthritis.org

Extract from the Versus Arthritis website.

"We are Versus Arthritis. We're the 10 million people living with arthritis. We're the carers, researchers, healthcare professionals, friends, parents, runners and fundraisers all united in our ambition to ensure that one day, no one will have to live with the pain, fatigue and isolation that arthritis causes.

Alongside volunteers, healthcare professionals, researchers and friends, we do everything we can to push back against arthritis. Together, we'll continue to develop breakthrough treatments, campaign relentlessly for arthritis to be seen as a priority, and support each other whenever we need it. Together, we're making real progress. But there's still a long way to go".

****

Chapter 12

Juvenile Idiopathic Arthritis

Juvenile idiopathic arthritis refers to a group of conditions involving joint inflammation that first appears before the age of 16. This condition is an autoimmune disorder, which means that the immune system malfunctions and attacks the body's organs and tissues, in this case the joints.

Researchers have described a number of types of juvenile idiopathic arthritis. The types are distinguished by their signs and symptoms, the number of joints affected, the results of laboratory tests, and the family history.

- *Systemic* juvenile idiopathic arthritis causes inflammation in one or more joints. A high daily fever that lasts at least 2 weeks either precedes or accompanies the arthritis. Individuals with systemic arthritis may also have a skin rash or enlargement of the lymph nodes (lymphadenopathy), liver (hepatomegaly), or spleen (splenomegaly).

- *Oligoarticular* juvenile idiopathic arthritis (also known as oligoarthritis) is marked by the occurrence of arthritis in four or fewer joints in the first 6 months of the disease. It is divided into two subtypes depending on the course of disease. If the arthritis is confined to four or fewer joints after 6 months, then the condition is classified as persistent oligoarthritis.

- If more than four joints are affected after 6 months, this condition is classified as extended oligoarthritis. Individuals with oligoarthritis are at increased risk of developing inflammation of the eye (uveitis).

- *Rheumatoid factor positive polyarticular juvenile idiopathic arthritis* (also known as polyarthritis, rheumatoid factor positive) causes inflammation in five or more joints within the first 6 months of the disease. Individuals with this condition also have a positive blood test for proteins called rheumatoid factors. This type of arthritis closely resembles rheumatoid arthritis as seen in adults.

- *Rheumatoid factor negative polyarticular juvenile idiopathic arthritis* (also known as polyarthritis, rheumatoid factor negative) is also characterized by arthritis in five or more joints within the first 6 months of the disease. Individuals with this type, however, test negative for rheumatoid factor in the blood.

- *Psoriatic juvenile idiopathic arthritis* involves arthritis that usually occurs in combination with a skin disorder called psoriasis. Psoriasis is a condition characterized by patches of red, irritated skin that are often covered by flaky white scales. Some affected individuals develop psoriasis before arthritis while others first develop arthritis. Other features of psoriatic arthritis include abnormalities of the fingers and nails or eye problems.

- *Enthesitis-related juvenile idiopathic arthritis* is characterized by tenderness where the bone meets a tendon, ligament, or other connective tissue.

127

- The most commonly affected places are the hips, knees, and feet. This tenderness, known as enthesitis, accompanies the joint inflammation of arthritis. Enthesitis-related arthritis may also involve inflammation in parts of the body other than the joints.

The last type of juvenile idiopathic arthritis is called *undifferentiated arthritis*. This classification is given to affected individuals who do not fit into any of the above types or who fulfil the criteria for more than one type of juvenile idiopathic arthritis.

Symptoms of JIA

Your child's JIA symptoms may take the form of occasional flare-ups or be continuous. These symptoms may include:

- Swollen, stiff and painful joints
- Decreased use of one or more particular joints
- Fatigue
- High fever and a characteristic rash (systemic onset JIA)
- Swollen lymph nodes (systemic onset JIA)
- Eye inflammation
- Decreased appetite, poor weight gain and slow growth

Causes

Juvenile idiopathic arthritis is thought to arise from a combination of genetic and environmental factors. The term "idiopathic" indicates that the specific cause of the disorder is unknown. Its signs and symptoms result from excessive inflammation in and around the joints. Inflammation occurs when the immune system sends signaling molecules and white blood cells to a site of injury or disease to fight microbial invaders and facilitate tissue repair. Normally, the body stops the inflammatory response after healing is complete to prevent damage to its own cells and tissues. In people with juvenile idiopathic arthritis, the inflammatory response is prolonged, particularly during joint movement. The reasons for this excessive inflammatory response are unclear.

Researchers have identified changes in several genes that may influence the risk of developing juvenile idiopathic arthritis. Some of these genes belong to a family of genes that provide instructions for making a group of related proteins called the human leukocyte antigen (HLA) complex. The HLA complex helps the immune system distinguish the body's own proteins from proteins made by foreign invaders (such as viruses and bacteria). Each HLA gene has many different normal variations, allowing each person's immune system to react to a wide range of foreign proteins. Certain normal variations of several HLA genes seem to affect the risk of developing juvenile idiopathic arthritis, and the specific type of the condition that a person may have.

Normal variations in several other genes have also been associated with juvenile idiopathic arthritis. Many of these genes are thought to play roles in immune system function. Additional unknown genetic influences and environmental factors, such as infection and other issues that affect immune health, are also likely to influence a person's chances of developing this complex disorder.

**

Inheritance factors

Most cases of juvenile idiopathic arthritis are sporadic, which means they occur in people with no history of the disorder in their family. A small percentage of cases of juvenile idiopathic arthritis have been reported to run in families, although the inheritance pattern of the condition is unclear. A sibling of a person with juvenile idiopathic arthritis has an estimated risk of developing the condition that is about 12 times that of the general population.

How is juvenile idiopathic arthritis treated?

The treatments for JIA aim to control the symptoms of the condition, enabling you to lead as active a life as possible. They also aim to reduce joint damage caused by the disease.

A number of different groups of medications are available. Painkillers might be useful, such as paracetamol or codeine. Some patients may be prescribed anti-inflammatories (NSAIDs) such as ibuprofen, naproxen or diclofenac, which work to reduce pain, stiffness and swelling of the joints.

Another group of medications, called disease modifying anti-rheumatic drugs (DMARDs) work by reducing inflammation in the joints, and helping to prevent long term joint damage. An example of a DMARD might be methotrexate, which is the one most commonly used in JIA. A newer group of drugs, called biologics, also work to reduce inflammation, and are used in cases of JIA that have not responded well to other therapies. Examples of biologics include etanercept, infliximab and adalimumab.

Organisations providing useful advice and support

JRIA at NRAS

www.jia.org.uk

Tel: 0845 458 3969

JRIA at NRAS aim to provide information and support for people affected by juvenile idiopathic arthritis (JIA) and rheumatoid arthritis (RA), their families, friends and carers, as well as health professionals.

JIA-at-NRAS is a part of the National Rheumatoid Arthritis Society (NRAS).

Versus Arthritis

www.versusarthritis.org

NHS

www.nhs.uk/Conditions/Arthritis

****

Chapter 13

The Importance of Exercise and Diet in Combating the Effects of Arthritis

---

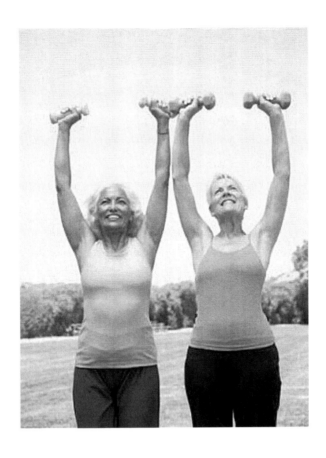

People with arthritis are encouraged to exercise regularly as it can assist pain control and reduces the risk of cardiovascular diseases. Also additional benefits of exercise include a healthier heart, better weight control and stress management.

The Importance of exercise

As well as strengthening the cardiovascular system and the body's muscles, many people exercise to keep fit, lose or maintain a healthy weight, sharpen their athletic skills, or purely for enjoyment. Regular, frequent physical exercise is recommended for people of all age groups as it boosts the immune system and helps to protect against conditions such as:

- Heart disease
- Stroke
- Type 2 diabetes
- Cancer and other major illnesses

In fact, it is known to cut your risk of major chronic illnesses/diseases by up to 50% and reduce your risk of early death by up to 30%. There are other health benefits of exercising on a regular basis which include:

- Improvements in mental health
- Better range of movement and joint mobility
- Stronger bones-which can help against osteoporosis
- Improved balance and co-ordination
- It boosts self-esteem/confidence
- It enhances sleep quality and energy levels
- It cuts risk of stress and depression

- It protects against dementia and alzheimer's disease
- Improved sleep
- Increased energy levels
- Better breathing

Defining exercise

In the UK, regular exercise is defined by the NHS as completing 150 minutes of moderate intensity aerobic activity a week. Aerobic activity at moderate intensity means exercising at a level that raises your heart rate and makes you sweat. This includes a multitude of sports. For example;

- Walking at a fast pace
- Jogging lightly
- Bike riding
- Rowing
- Playing tennis or badminton
- Water aerobics

Obviously, depending on what type of arthritis you have, not all of the above exercises will be suitable for you. However, the less time you spend sitting down, the better it will be for your health. Sedentary behaviour, such as sitting or lying down for long periods, increases your risk of weight gain and obesity, which in turn, may also up your risk of chronic diseases such as heart disease.

Outlined below are a few tips to help you on your way to a fulfilling exercise regime.

Beginning a new exercise routine

During the first few weeks of a new exercise routine you can expect to feel a small increase in levels of discomfort because you are awakening muscles that are not used to it. Don't overdo it as this can result in fatigue and joint swelling. If you are working with a physiotherapist they will advise you on appropriate levels of exercise.

The importance of good posture

If you have arthritis, you will find that developing and maintaining good posture can really help to put less strain on your body. Poor posture can develop for a number of reasons, but it can be due to muscles and tendons being either too tight or too weak and not supporting the body as they should.

Exercise is key to maintaining good posture, and different exercises can help in different ways, including to strengthen, lengthen and even shorten muscles. Below are a few tips for achieving good posture when standing:

- Stand with your feet slightly apart

- Gently lengthen and straighten your neck and back, allow your shoulders to relax and drop allowing your chin to relax

- Your arms should be relaxed and hanging loose

- Very gently tilt your pelvis slightly, so that it is level: this will encourage your stomach to flatten and your bottom to tuck under

- Your hips should be in line with your knees and feet

You should check your posture by looking in a mirror. Think about posture as you go through the day, by doing this you will increase your body awareness.

Exercising after having a joint replacement

If you are awaiting joint replacement surgery such as hips, knees or shoulders (which may have been the result of arthritis) it is important that you exercise as much as possible beforehand as this will help to strengthen the muscles around the joint that is being replaced. This will help to speed up the recovery after the operation. The hospital will advise you on different exercises.

After the surgery, you should receive advice on the correct techniques when exercising. Low impact exercises such as swimming and walking are ideal but it is important not to overdo it.

More strenuous exercises such as running should be avoided after surgery in order to avoid damaging a joint. Also, it is important to avoid any activity that can lead to dislocation of a joint. For example, after a hip replacement avoid excessive bending or lifting your knee higher than hip height.

Flare ups and exercising

As we discussed in earlier chapters, some people with forms of arthritis such as rheumatoid arthritis or lupus experience flare ups. This is when the inflammation of a joint or joints becomes suddenly active.

Be very gentle and adopt mild exercises if flare up happens.

Different types of exercises

It is a known fact that people with arthritis benefit from a range of different movement, strengthening and aerobic exercises. A good exercise program will include all three types of exercise.

Range of movement exercises

Range of movement exercises are exercises that are given for a specific joint where there is a decreased amount of movement. These exercises can be assisted by gravity, assisted by yourself (e.g. the movement is performed to the achievable range, and then additional pressure is applied by another part of the body such as your hands to achieve a greater range), assisted by another person, done within water and assisted by an external machine.

There are many benefits of seeing a physiotherapist if movement is reduced at a joint. Range of movement exercises can:

- Increase movement at a joint
- Increase the function of a joint and the whole limb
- Improve movement efficiency
- Increase independence
- Decrease pain
- Improve and maintain joint integrity

These benefits can have a positive effect on your life if you are suffering from decreased range of movement at a joint. These particular exercises are important and should be carried out as frequently as possible.

Strengthening/flexibility/balance exercises

These exercises are recommended to help stiffness and pain, particularly hips and knees. They work on strengthening muscles, which in turn helps to support joints more effectively. Below are some basic exercises which consist of a range of sitting, flexibility and balance exercises which are easy to carry out can be done in the home and which will greatly enhance your overall well being.

Aerobic exercises

These are more vigorous exercises and make you breath faster which raises your heart rate. Examples include walking, swimming and cycling. The aim should be to complete around 30 minutes of this type of exercise per week.

Examples of aerobic exercises

- Walking
- Swimming and Hydrotherapy
- Aqua aerobics
- Dance
- Cycling
- Attending a gym or leisure centre-Exercise classes

Other forms of exercise

The exercises below are also useful for exercising the joints and muscles.

- Yoga and Pilates
- Tai Chi

You can find out more about these types of exercise by visiting your local leisure centre or contacting your local branch of arthritis care.

Arthritis Care at arthritiscare.org.uk have a whole range of illustrated exercises covering range of movement, strengthening and aerobic exercises.

In addition, The NHS website www.nhs.uk/live-well/exercise/strength-and-flex-exercise-plan has a comprehensive range of illustrated exercises for arthritis sufferers and covers a whole range of Strength, Flexibility and Balance exercises.

Arthritis Care also has some very useful tips for specific types of arthritis, listed throughout this book. As we have seen, the types of exercise that you can do will be very much dictated by the type of condition you have.

****

Arthritis and diet

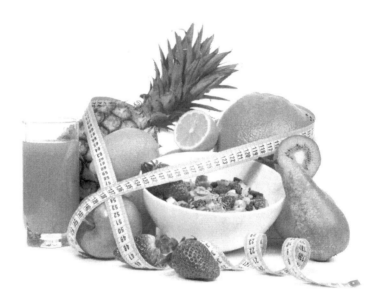

It is a fact that eating well is important, whether or not a person has arthritis. The foods you choose to eat in your daily diet make a difference not only to managing arthritis, but also to how well you feel and how much energy you have every day. How much you need to eat and drink is based on your age, gender, how active you are and the goals you are looking to achieve.

Portion sizes have grown in recent years, as the plates and bowls we use have got bigger. Use smaller crockery to cut back on your portion sizes, while making the food on your plate look bigger. No single food contains all the essential nutrients you need in the right proportion. That's why you need to consume foods from each of the main food groups to eat well.

The advice given below is general but will benefit those with arthritis and joint pain.

Fruit and vegetables

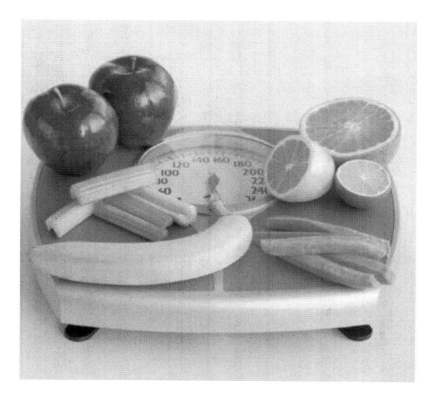

Naturally low in fat and calories and packed full of vitamins, minerals and fibre, fruit and vegetables add flavour and variety to every meal. They may also help protect against stroke, heart disease, high blood pressure and some cancers.

Everyone should eat at least five portions a day. Fresh, frozen, dried and canned fruit in juice and canned vegetables in water all count. Go for a rainbow of colours to get as wide a range of vitamins and minerals as possible.

Starchy foods

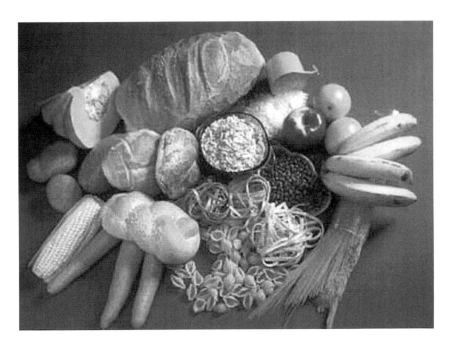

Potatoes, rice, pasta, bread, chapattis, naan and plantain all contain carbohydrate, which is broken down into glucose and used by your cells as fuel.

Better options of starchy foods – such as wholegrain bread, wholewheat pasta and basmati, brown or wild rice – contain more fibre, which helps to keep your digestive system working well. They are generally more slowly absorbed (that is, they have a lower glycaemic index, or GI), keeping you feeling fuller for longer. Try to include some starchy foods every day.

Fish, meat, eggs and nuts.

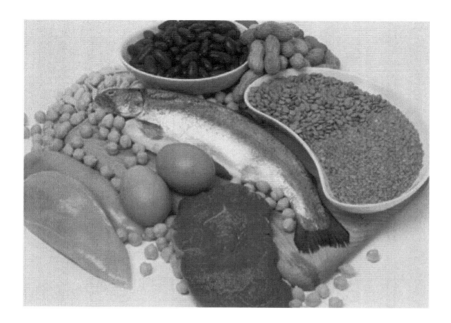

These foods are high in protein, which helps with building and replacing muscles. They contain minerals, such as iron, which are vital for producing red blood cells. Oily fish, such as mackerel, salmon and sardines, also provide omega-3, which can help protect the heart. Beans, pulses, soya and tofu are also good sources of protein.

Aim to have some food from this group every day, with at least 1–2 portions of oily fish a week.

Dairy foods

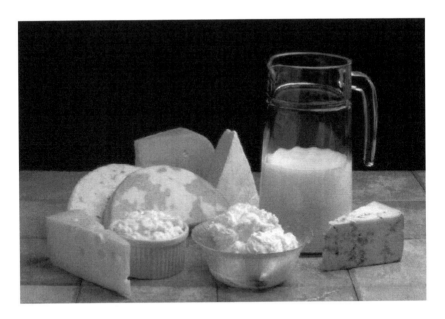

Milk, cheese and yogurt contain calcium, which is vital as it keeps bones and teeth strong. They're good sources of protein, too.

Some dairy foods are high in fat, particularly saturated fat, so choose lower-fat alternatives (check for added sugar, though). Semi-skimmed milk actually contains more calcium than whole milk. Aim to have some dairy every day, but don't overdo it.

Foods high in fat and sugar

You can enjoy food from this group as an occasional treat in a balanced diet, but remember that sugary foods and drinks will add extra calories – and sugary drinks will raise blood glucose – so opt for diet/light or low-calorie alternatives. Or choose water – it's calorie free! Fat is high in calories, so try to reduce the amount of oil or butter you use in cooking. Remember to use unsaturated oils, such as sunflower, rapeseed or olive oil, as these types are better for your heart.

Salt

Too much salt can make you more at risk of high blood pressure and stroke. Processed foods can be very high in salt. Try cooking more meals from scratch at home, where you can control the amount of salt you use – when there are so many delicious spices in your kitchen, you really can enjoy your favourite recipes with less salt.

Adults should have no more than 1 tsp (6g) of salt a day, while children have even lower targets.

Natural remedies and Arthritis

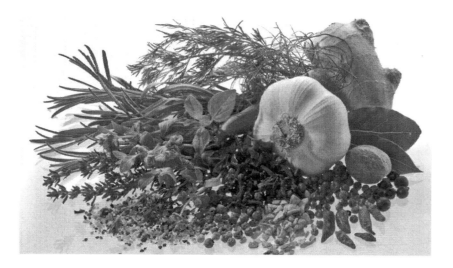

Many common herbs and spices are claimed to have properties that make them useful for people with arthrits.

A number of clinical studies have been carried out in recent years that show potential links between herbal therapies and improved health which has led to an increase in people with arthritis using these more 'natural' ingredients to help manage their condition. Plant-based therapies that have been shown in some studies to have beneficial effects include:

- Aloe vera
- Bilberry extract
- Bitter melon
- Cinnamon
- Fenugreek
- Ginger
- Okra

If you decide to follow a particular dietary path then it is important that you first discuss this with your doctor.

Below are listed 10 types of foods which are seen to have beneficial effects for those with arthritis.

Fortunately, there are many foods that can ease inflammation and may help relieve some of the joint pain associated with arthritis. The below are ten types of food that can be particularly beneficial.

1. Fatty Fish

Fatty fish varieties such as salmon, mackerel, sardines and trout are high in omega-3 fatty acids, which have been shown to have potent anti-inflammatory effects.

Fish is also a good source of vitamin D, which can help prevent deficiency. Multiple studies have found that rheumatoid arthritis may be associated with low levels of vitamin D, which could contribute to symptoms

It is recommended that you should include at least two servings of fatty fish in your diet each week to take advantage of the beneficial anti-inflammatory properties.

2. Garlic

Garlic is jam-packed with health benefits and has been shown to have an anti-inflammatory effect that may help decrease symptoms of arthritis.

In one study, researchers analyzed the diets of 1,082 twins. They found that those who ate more garlic had a reduced risk of hip osteoarthritis, likely thanks to garlic's strong anti-inflammatory properties.

Another test-tube study showed that a specific component in garlic could decrease some of the inflammatory markers associated with arthritis. Adding garlic to your diet could benefit both arthritis symptoms and overall health.

3. Ginger

Besides adding a burst of flavor to teas, soups and sweets, ginger may also help ease the symptoms of arthritis.

A 2001 study assessed the effects of ginger extract in 261 patients with osteoarthritis of the knee. After six weeks, 63% of participants experienced improvements in knee pain. One test-tube study also found that ginger and its components blocked the production of substances that promote inflammation in the body.

Consuming ginger in fresh, powdered or dried form may reduce inflammation and aid in reducing symptoms of arthritis.

4. Broccoli

It's no secret that broccoli is one of the healthiest foods out there. In fact, it may even be associated with reduced inflammation.One study that looked at the diets of 1,005 women found that the intake of cruciferous vegetables like broccoli was associated with decreased levels of inflammatory markers.

Broccoli also contains important components that could help reduce symptoms of arthritis. For example, sulforaphane is a compound found in broccoli. Test-tube studies have shown that it blocks the formation of a type of cell involved in rheumatoid arthritis development.

5. Walnuts

Walnuts are nutrient-dense and loaded with compounds that may help reduce the inflammation associated with joint disease.

Walnuts are especially high in omega-3 fatty acids, which have been shown to decrease the symptoms of arthritis. In one study, 90 patients with rheumatoid arthritis took supplements of either omega-3 fatty acids or olive oil.

6. Berries

Tons of antioxidants, vitamins and minerals are crammed into each serving of berries, which may partially account for their unique ability to decrease inflammation.

Berries are rich in quercetin and rutin, two plant compounds that boast a huge number of benefits for your health.

There is a wide variety of berries to choose from. Strawberries, blackberries and blueberries are just a few options that can satisfy your sweet tooth and provide plenty of arthritis-fighting nutrients.

7. Spinach

Leafy greens like spinach are full of nutrients, and some of their components may actually be able to help decrease inflammation caused by arthritis.

Spinach, in particular, contains plenty of antioxidants as well as plant compounds that can relieve inflammation and help fight disease.

Spinach is especially high in the antioxidant kaempferol, which has been shown to decrease the effects of the inflammatory agents associated with rheumatoid arthritis.

8. Grapes

Grapes are nutrient-dense, high in antioxidants and possess inflammatory properties.

Grapes contain several compounds that have been shown to be beneficial in the treatment of arthritis. For example, resveratrol is an antioxidant present in the skin of grapes. Grapes also contain a plant compound called proanthocyanidin, which may have promising effects on arthritis.

9. Olive Oil

Well-known for its anti-inflammatory properties, olive oil may have a favorable effect on arthritis symptoms.

Although more research is needed on the effects of olive oil on arthritis, including olive oil and other healthy fats in your diet can definitely benefit your health, and may also reduce arthritis symptoms.

10. Tart Cherry Juice

Tart cherry juice is an increasingly popular beverage derived from the fruit of the *Prunus cerasus* tree. This potent juice offers a wide array of nutrients and health benefits, and may even help reduce the symptoms of arthritis.

Be sure to look for an unsweetened variety of tart cherry juice to make sure you don't consume excess added sugar. In combination with a healthy diet and other arthritis-fighting foods, a serving of unsweetened tart cherry juice per day may help decrease some of the symptoms of arthritis.

In summary:

It's clear that diet can play a major role in arthritis severity and symptoms. Luckily, a variety of foods with powerful components may offer relief from inflammation and arthritis — while also promoting overall health.

Along with conventional treatments, eating a nutritious diet containing healthy fats, a few servings of fatty fish and plenty of produce may help reduce some symptoms of arthritis.

**

Organisations providing useful advice and support

Exercising

Arthritis Care (Versus Arthritis)

There are Living with Arthritis services all over the country, often run by people who have arthritis who can help you to understand your condition and manage your symptoms better and talk through your options. There are Arthritis Care groups and branches, run by people with arthritis, giving you the opportunity to spend time with others who share and understand what it's like to live with arthritis.

Or you may prefer to visit their online community where you can chat to others with arthritis about the things that matter to you. To find out more go to: arthritiscare.org.uk, call the free helpline weekdays on 0808 800 4050 or contact one of their offices:

- England: 020 7380 6540
- Northern Ireland : 028 9078 2940
- Scotland: 0141 954 7776
- Wales: 029 2044 4155

General

Sport England

Tel: 0345 850 8508

sportengland.org

English Federation of Disability Sport

Tel: 01509 227750 or 0161 228 2868

efds.co.uk

Sport Wales

Tel: 0300 300 3111

sportwales.org.uk

Disability Sport Wales

Tel: 0300 300 3115

disabilitysportwales.com

Sport Northern Ireland

Tel: 028 9038 1222

sportni.net

Disability Sports Northern Ireland

Tel: 028 9046 9925

disni.co.uk

Sport Scotland

Tel: 0141 634 6500

sportscotland.org.uk

Scottish Disability Sport

Tel: 0131 317 1130

scottishdisabilityport.com

Other useful organisations

Classes and trainers

Contact your local council, sports centre or libraries, or check online for details of exercise and sports clubs and courses available in your area.

Excel 2000

Offers disabled people structured movement to music workshops as well as video and audio tapes.
Tel: 01263 825670
excel2000.org.uk

Extend

Movement to music for the over 60speople of any age.
Tel: 01582 832760
extend.org.uk

The Fitness League

Offers low-impact exercise by trained teachers in a class situation. Classes are suitable for all ages and abilities.
Tel: 01403 266000
thefitnessleague.com

The National Register of Personal

Trainers

Can provide details of registered trainers in your area.
Tel: 01536 425920
nrpt.co.uk

Sports Coach UK
An organisation of coaches for all sports.
Tel: 0113 274 4802
sportscoachuk.org

The YMCAfit
Offers courses across the UK.
Tel: 020 7343 1850
ymcafit.org.uk

Alexander Technique
The Society of Teachers of the
Alexander Technique
The largest regulatory body of Alexander Technique teachers.
Tel: 020 8885 6524
alexandertechnique.co.uk

Cycling
British Cycling
Tel: 0161 274 2000
britishcycling.org.uk

Pilates
Body Control Pilates
A list of UK instructors is available on their website.
Tel: 020 7636 8900
bodycontrolpilates.com

Swimming
National Association of Swimming
Clubs for the Handicapped
Tel: 01329 833689
nasch.org.uk

Tai Chi
Tai Chi Union for Great Britain. Has a list of registered Tai Chi Union instructors throughout the UK (details online).
Tel: 01403 257918
taichiunion.com

Walking
The British Walking Federation
Promotes non-competitive sports for health and international relations. It has contact details of walking clubs around the UK.
bwf-ivv.org.uk

Yoga
The British Wheel of Yoga
The governing body of yoga.
Tel: 01529 306851
bwy.org.uk

Other exercise
Rebounding
Low-impact action on small trampolines to strengthen with minimal impact.
Tel: 01252 883 871
rebound-uk.com

Aqua Fitness/Aqua Jogging/
Aqua Zumba
www.zumba.com

Dietary Advice

Arthritis Care (Versus Arthritis)
arthritiscare.org.uk

UK offices:

- England: 020 7380 6500
- Northern Ireland : 028 9078 2940
- Scotland: 0141 954 7776
- Wales: 029 2044 4155

British Dietetic Association
5th Floor Charles House
148/149 Great Charles Street
Queensway
Birmingham
B3 3HT
0121 200 8080
www.bda.uk.com

Food Standards Agency
Aviation House
125 Kingsway
London

WC2B 6NH

020 7276 8829

www.food.gov.uk

NHS Direct

0845 4647

www.nhsdirect.nhs.uk

Vegetarian Society

Parkdale

Durham Road

Altrincham

Cheshire

WA14 4QG

0161 925 2000

www.vegcoc.org

Websites

Healthline

www.healthline.com/health/foods-to-avoid-with-arthritis

NHS

Diet

www.nhs.uk/conditions/arthritis/living-with

Arthritis.org

www.arthritis.org/living-with-arthritis/arthritis-diet/best-food

There are numerous other websites dealing with arthritis, many saying the same things.

NHS Wales
One of the best diet sheets can be found at NHS Wales. This is a comprehensive overview of dietary related issues as they affect arthritis sufferers. there is a very useful downloadable PDF.

www.wales.nhs.uk/Diet-and-arthritis

****

Acupressure, 33

Acupuncture, 33, 80

Aerobic activity, 134

Aerobic exercise, 27, 54

Aloe vera, 146

Alzheimer's disease, 134

Analgesics, 28

Ankylosing spondylitis, 6, 11, 51, 52

Antibiotics, 114

Anticonvulsants, 79

Antipsychotics, 79

Arthritis Care, 34, 117, 139, 151, 156

Assistive Devices, 32

Auto-immune condition, 9, 12, 13

Back pain, 18

Badminton, 134

Bike riding, 134

Bilberry extract, 146

Biological treatments, 44, 106, 107

Bitter melon, 146

Bone spurs, 63

British Association of Dermatologists, 103

Calcium crystal diseases, 13

Cancer, 133

Capsaicin cream, 29

Cardiovascular diseases, 133

Carpal tunnel syndrome, 46

Cartilage, 8, 22
Cervical myelopathy, 46
Cervical spondylitis, 6, 11
Cheese, 144
Chemical imbalances, 75
Chronic Fatigue Syndrome, 76
Cinnamon, 146
Codeine, 29, 68
Cognitive behavioural therapy, 72, 79
Cognitive problems ('fibro-fog'), 73
Complementary therapies, 107
Corticosteroids, 29, 55, 105
Cryotherapy, 31
Cutaneous lupus, 85
Cycling, 19, 138

Dairy foods, 144
Dehydrated spinal discs., 63
Dementia, 134
Depression, 133
Depression, 74
Diabetes, 25
Disease-modifying anti-rheumatic drugs (DMARDs), 43, 104, 112, 114
Dopamine, 75
Drug-induced lupus. (DILE), 85

Endorphins, 19
Enteropathic arthritis, 3, 6, 51, 58, 59, 60
Entheses, 11

Exercise, 132
Eye pain, 14, 110, 113

Fat, 144
Fenugreek, 146
Fibromyalgia, 3, 6, 12, 71, 73, 75, 77, 83
Fish, 143
Flare ups, 136

Genes, 7, 13, 23, 57, 75, 129
Genetics, 75, 87
Genital tract, 14, 110
Giant Cell Arteritis (GCA)., 15
Ginger, 146
Gout, 3, 5, 6, 13, 94, 95

Hands, 9, 12, 29, 30, 37, 74, 102, 113, 120, 137
Heart disease, 133
Heart Disease, 25
Herbs, 145
Herniated discs, 63
Hips, 9, 14, 22, 24, 28, 33, 52, 110, 112, 118, 119, 127, 135, 136, 138
Hyaluronic acid, 29
Hyperuricaemia, 95

Immune system, 9, 10, 12, 13, 16, 33, 38, 43, 45, 56, 84, 90, 103, 106, 111, 120, 122, 126, 128, 129, 133
Iritis, 14, 110, 113
Iron, 143

Jogging, 134
Joint, 8, 12, 26, 33, 41, 112
joint pain, 7, 86, 99, 112, 115, 141, 146
Juvenile idiopathic arthritis (JIA), 6, 16

Kidney stones, 98
Knee ligament, 15
knees, 8, 9, 13, 14, 22, 24, 28, 29, 33, 52, 95, 102, 110, 112, 127, 135, 136, 138
Ligaments, 8
Lupus, 3, 6, 12, 84, 92

Magnetic resonance imaging (MRI), 27
Manual therapy, 32
Massage, 33, 80
Muscle relaxants, 78

Narcotic pain relievers, 25
Natural remedies, 145
Neonatal lupus, 86
NHS, 134
Nonsteroidal anti-inflammatory drugs (NSAIDs, 28, 122

Obesity, 23, 25, 97, 134
Okra, 146
Oligoarthritis, 126
Oligoarticular juvenile idiopathic arthritis, 126
Omega-3, 143
Opioids, 29
Osteoarthritis, 3, 5, 6, 9, 22, 23, 27, 34

Paracetamol, 29, 55, 67, 68, 77, 130

Pilates, 19, 138, 154

Plant-based therapies, 146

Platelet rich plasma (PRP, 31

Polyarthritis, 127

Polymyalgia rheumatica, 6, 14, 118

Potatoes, 142

Prednisolone, 68, 121, 122

Primary hyperurcaemia, 95

Processed foods, 145

Protein, 143, 144

Psoriatic arthritis, 6, 13, 101

Pulses, 143

Reactive arthritis, 6, 14, 110, 112, 113

Red blood cells, 143

Repetitive microtrauma, 15

Rheumatoid arthritis, 6, 9, 10, 37, 46, 47, 50

Rowing, 134

Salt, 145

Secondary arthritis, 15

Secondary hyperuricaemia, 95

Sedentary behaviour, 134

Semi-skimmed milk, 144

Serotonin, 75, 78

Sexually transmitted infection, 14, 110, 111

Sleep quality, 133

Soya, 143

Spices, 145

Spondylosis, 11
Starchy foods, 142
Steroid injections, 30
Steroids, 30, 114
Stress management, 133
Stretching, 28
Stroke, 133
Swimming, 19, 49, 138, 155
Systemic juvenile idiopathic arthritis, 126

Tai Chi, 19, 138, 155
Temporal arteritis, 119, 123
Tendinopathy, 18
Tendon rupture, 46
Tennis, 134
The National Institute for Health and Care Excellence (NICE), 43, 56
Thermotherapy, 31
Tofu, 143
Tophaceous gout, 98
Tophi, 99
Tramadol, 28, 29, 77
Transcutaneous electrical nerve stimulation (TENS), 31
Trycyclic anti-depressants, 68
Tuberculosis, 45

Undifferentiated arthritis, 128
Uric acid arthropathy, 94

Vasculitis, 46

Vegetables, 141

Water aerobics, 134
Weight Management, 28

Yoga,, 19, 91
Yogurt, 144

****